FAMILIAL POLYPOSIS COLI

FAMILIAL POLYPOSIS COLI

Family studies,
histopathology,
differential diagnosis,
and
results of treatment

H. J. R. Bussey

The Johns Hopkins University Press
Baltimore and London

The Johns Hopkins University Press, Baltimore, Maryland 21218
The Johns Hopkins University Press Ltd., London

Library of Congress Catalog Card Number 74–24392
ISBN 0–8018–1686–6

Library of Congress Cataloging in Publication Data

Bussey, H   J   R
    Familial polyposis coli.

    Based on the author's thesis, University of
London, 1970
    Bibliography: pp. 95–102
    Includes index.
    1. Intestinal polyps—Genetic aspects.
I. Title. [DNLM: 1. Colonic neoplasms—
Familial and genetic. 2. Intestinal polyps—
Familial and genetic. WI520 B981f]
RC280.I8B86   616.9'92'347   74–24392
ISBN 0–8018–1686–6

H. J. R. Bussey, O.B.E., B.Sc., Ph.D.,
is senior research fellow
at St. Mark's Hospital in London.

contents

preface

Since its earliest reports adenomatous polyposis coli has fascinated clinicians concerned with disease of the large intestine. With its frequent onset in youth, its often fatal outcome, and its familial character, the disease presents a picture of doom, sinister and inevitable as that of any fiction story of a family curse. Advances in medicine, particularly in the field of surgery, have spared the victims the worst effects of the curse, although this still awaits a final exorcism.

Interesting though the study of polyposis coli as a disease entity may be, its main value probably lies in the light that its investigation may throw on the much wider problem of the nature and development of intestinal adenomas when these are solitary or few in number. All available evidence suggests that little, if any, distinction can be made between adenomas occurring by the hundreds, as in polyposis, or as isolated tumors. The two conditions, at first sight so dissimilar, may both be due to changes in the intestinal mucosa differing in degree rather than in nature. This possibility would be greatly strengthened if the hypothesis advanced in 1965 by Professor A. M. O. Veale proves to be correct. He suggested that not only are the adenomas of polyposis the result of inheritance or genetic mutation but that all adenomas of the large intestine have a genetic origin, and on this basis he constructed a genetic model to account for the known facts. So far relatively little research has been undertaken into the genetic aspects of intestinal tumors, but the results tend to support the hypothesis rather than disprove it.

It would be a matter of considerable importance if it could be shown that fundamentally the same factors are responsible for both multiple and isolated adenomas. There is no doubt that polyposis cases provide better facilities for the observation and analysis of these factors than do patients with isolated adenomas. The use of polyposis coli as a model for the study of the histological, enzymic, and other biochemical changes occurring in both the early and late stages of adenoma formation could be of immense value. Isolated adenomatous tumors are mature lesions when found on clinical examination, even when discovered accidentally. It has not been possible to observe the mode of origin and the intermediate stages of growth before a definite polyp is already formed. On the other hand, any colectomy specimen removed for polyposis shows numerous examples of all stages of adenoma formation. Also the study of polyposis families might indicate the possible interaction of environmental and genetic factors.

That there exists a relationship between adenomas and carcinomas of the large intestine becomes increasingly certain. In fact, it is probable that most, possibly even all, carcinomas arise in preexisting adenomatous tumors. One method of controlling intestinal cancer could be by attacking its precursor—the adenoma. It has already been suggested that the investigation of the origin and behavior of adenomatous tumors is most easily carried out in the patient with polyposis. Success in the control of adenomas would benefit both those with polyposis coli and those individuals in the general population with isolated adenomas, but to greatly differing degrees in their overall value. Against the 40 to 50 individuals with polyposis estimated to be born each year in the United Kingdom must be set the 15,000 persons who die annually from cancer of the colon and rectum. It is the possibility of helping so many that justifies a study in depth of the few suffering from a rare condition like adenomatous polyposis coli.

This study could not have been undertaken over the long period of time necessary for genetic observations without the generous financial help given for the past half-century by the Cancer Research Campaign (formerly the British Empire Cancer Campaign).

To Dr. Cuthbert Dukes belongs the credit for initiating the St. Mark's Hospital Polyposis Register and with it the systematic investigation of polyposis coli. I acknowledge gratefully the help and encouragement I had, not only from him, in continuing this work but also from his successor as director of the Research Department, Dr. B. C. Morson. This work has only been possible with the continued support of the consultant staff at St. Mark's Hospital in allowing me access to their patients and records and with the help received from many clinicians and pathologists throughout the country who have supplied clinical histories and histological material.

My thanks are also due to Lloyd Soodeen for his cooperation in preparing the histology slides, to Norman Mackie for the help with the illustrations and to Dorinda Harwood for secretarial assistance.

This monograph is a continuation and elaboration of work submitted in 1970 for the degree of Ph.D. at the University of London.

glossary

Polyp	Macroscopic descriptive term for a pedunculated or semipedunculated tumor attached to the mucosal surface. Its general use for any mass of tissue projecting into the bowel lumen, i.e., synonymous with 'tumor' is not favored and it should not be used as synonymous with 'adenoma'.
Polyposis	A condition in which an unspecific number of polyps are present in the large intestine.
Adenomatous polyposis coli	Also known as polyposis coli, familial polyposis, multiple polyposis, multiple adenomatosis. An inheritable condition in which the large intestine contains multiple adenomas, multiple being defined as more than 100.
Polyposis family	A family with at least one member suffering from polyposis.
Polyposis coli family	A family in which at least one member suffers from adenomatous polyposis coli.
Polyposis coli patient	**a)** Patient suffering from adenomatous polyposis coli. **b)** Parent, sibling, or child of (a) known to have multiple polyps or carcinoma of the large intestine, or both.

	c) Individual without evidence of having adenomas or carcinoma of the large intestine whose parent or sibling had adenomatous polyposis coli and who has transmitted the disease to his or her children.
Polyposis coli family members	Considered to be those individuals who have adenomatous polyposis coli, together with their brothers and sisters and the children of affected members, i.e., all those with the disease or at risk of inheriting it. The children of unaffected members are not at risk.
Propositus polyposis patient	Patient presenting because of symptoms due to polyposis coli.
"Call-up" family member	Family member at risk who accepts an invitation to be examined.
Adenoma	A benign neoplastic tumor arising from intestinal mucus-secreting epithelium and showing varying degrees of atypia.
Tubular adenoma	Adenoma composed of branching tubules embedded in lamina propria.
Villous adenoma	Adenoma composed of finger-like processes, usually with pointed ends, consisting of thin strands of stroma covered by epithelium.
Carcinoma in-situ	A term sometimes used to describe areas in neoplastic epithelial tumors where there is severe dysplasia and atypia, similar to that seen in adenocarcinoma and from which they may only be distinguished by the absence of invasion of subjacent tissues.
	The policy at St. Mark's Hospital is not to use this term, but to describe such growths as adenomas showing severe dysplasia but no invasive carcinoma and to regard them as clinically benign.
Adenocarcinoma	A neoplastic epithelial tumor with varying degrees of dysplasia which has invaded across the line of the muscularis mucosae.
Hyperplastic polyp	Synonymous with "metaplastic" polyp.

Metaplastic polyp   A non-neoplastic lesion arising from epithelium of the colon or rectum. The tubules are increased in length, with hyperplasia of the epithelium in the lower part of the tubules, and there is uneven cell size and depletion of goblet cells in the upper part. Cystic dilatation of the tubules is common.

FAMILIAL POLYPOSIS COLI

1
introduction

During the last 250 years a heterogenous mass of material has accumulated under the term "intestinal polyposis," and the classification of this material into separate entities began about eighty years ago and is still proceeding. The first report of a condition of multiple polyps in the large bowel is usually ascribed to Menzel (1721), and it is almost certain that the case he described was one of inflammatory polyposis. Another century was to elapse before further cases were reported (Wagner 1832; Rokitansky 1839; Lebert 1861; Luschka 1861). Most of these earlier cases were probably also inflammatory in origin, or to use the term suggested for them by Virchow (1863), "colitis polyposa." Corvisart (1847) may have given the first record of a case of adenomatous polyposis and Chargelaigue (1859) probably gave the first definite account of the disease which he found in a 16-year-old girl and a man of 21 years. Woodward (1881) divided polyposis cases into primary polyposis, that is to say, adenomatous polyposis, and secondary polyposis which followed inflammation of the intestine. The growing science of histology helped in this differentiation by demonstrating microscopically that the polyps of the primary type were hyperplastic or neoplastic in nature and those of the secondary class were inflammatory. The distinction was more firmly established when a familial tendency was observed in the primary type of polyposis. Cripps (1882) first recorded polyposis coli in two members of the same family who were brother and sister. This was followed by other reports of the familial nature of the disease (Bickersteth 1890; Niemack 1902; Zahlmann 1903), which was recognized by the more general use of the term "familial polyposis coli." The association of the disease with cancer of the large intestine appears to have been mentioned first by Handford (1890), and during the next thirty years both the precancerous nature and the hereditary character of the lesion had been firmly established.

By the beginning of the century there was a general tendency to divide polyposis cases into familial and nonfamilial types, these corresponding approximately with familial adenomatosis and inflammatory polyposis (colitis polyposa) respectively. The differential diagnosis of adenomatosis and other forms of intestinal polyposis is dealt with later, but it may be stated here that neither of the two types was pure. From the familial type a second group was separated following reports by Peutz (1921) and Jeghers and his co-workers (1949). Although most of the nonfamilial conditions appeared to be sequelae to previous inflammation of the bowel, other causes, such as schistosomiasis, were discovered. Moreover, polyposis due to environmental factors, such as bacteria or parasites, could occur with a familial tendency not due to genetic inheritance. More accurate clinical, histological, and genetic observations on the various forms of intestinal polyposis have been made in the past fifty years and have done much to clarify the subject, particularly in regard to familial adenomatosis.

One factor responsible for this improvement was the establishment at St. Mark's Hospital of a polyposis register. Three families were investigated by Lockhart-Mummery (1925) at St. Mark's Hospital, and these, together with 10 families from the literature, were reviewed by Dukes (1930). The 3 families formed the nucleus of the St. Mark's Hospital Polyposis Register, which by 1952 had grown to 42 families, forming the basis of a detailed survey of the clinicopathological features of the disease (Dukes 1952). The Register now contains records of 294 families with gastrointestinal polyposis, 200 of which are of the adenomatous type. The operation of this Register will be explained in Chapter 2. It is probably the largest collection of polyposis cases existing and is still being added to at the rate of a new family every month.

The St. Mark's Hospital material was also used in a genetic study by Veale (1965), in which he suggested that the gene responsible for the classical form of polyposis might be modified by another gene, also a cause of adenoma production, and that the combination of the two genes could cause earlier and more severe adenomatous polyposis. It is now suggested that this second gene, which ordinarily produces only solitary or few adenomas, can occasionally cause polyps in sufficient numbers to be mistaken for classical polyposis. Unless further research proves the contrary, such cases should not be included under the classification of polyposis coli.

At about the same time that Dukes published his survey of the disease in 1952, Gardner and his co-workers described the syndrome that now bears his name (Gardner 1951; Gardner & Plenk 1952; Gardner & Richards 1953). New cases of Gardner's syndrome have been constantly added, and the subject has acquired an extensive literature and provoked considerable discussion on what constitutes the syndrome and what its clinical and genetic relationship is to ordinary polyposis coli.

Other conditions formerly believed to be polyposis coli have also been recognized as different lesions. The first of these was the Peutz–Jeghers syndrome. Peutz (1921) reported a remarkable family, members of which suffered from multiple intestinal polyps, the affected persons also having a curious pigmentation of the lips and buccal membrane. Previous reference to similar familial pigmentation had been made (Hutchinson 1896), but its significance was not appreciated until Jeghers and his colleagues reported a series of cases in 1949. The earlier reports stressed a high cancer incidence, but it was later shown that not only was this due to mistaken pathological interpretation but also that the polyps themselves were not adenomatous but hamartomatous in nature (Dormandy 1957; Bartholomew & Dahlin 1958; Rintala 1959; Morson 1962).

Recently, it has been found that some cases included in the records as adenomatosis were, in fact, not adenomatous in nature. These cases of nonadenomatous polyposis fell into two categories. The first group of "contaminants" was discovered when a survey of the age distribution of adenomas of the large intestine revealed that even in polyposis coli the adenomas rarely appeared before the age of 10 years and seldom gave rise to symptoms before 15 years. This led to a review of the younger members in the register, particularly two, who at the ages of 9 and 13 had presented with rectal symptoms. In both cases the polyps were found to be juvenile polyps (mucous retention polyps) and not adenomas (Veale, McColl, Bussey, & Morson 1966). These tumors, like the Peutz–Jeghers polyps, are hamartomatous in character (Morson 1962b). Since in some instances more than one member of the family is known to suffer from multiple juvenile polyposis, and since a possible genetic relationship to adenomatosis may exist, a mistaken diagnosis of polyposis coli was easily made.

The recognition of multiple juvenile polyposis emphasized the necessity to base the diagnosis of any case of polyposis on histology whenever possible. The sections of cases in the register were reviewed and every effort was made to obtain sections where these had not been previously available. One result of this survey was the appearance of a further type of nonadenomatous polyposis. This is multiple metaplastic polyposis, in which multiple polyps, having the histology of "hyperplastic" polyps (Westhues 1934) or, as they have more recently been termed (Morson 1962a), "metaplastic" polyps, are found in the large intestine and are occasionally sufficiently large and numerous to cause confusion in diagnosis.

Benign lymphoid hyperplasia, probably as the result of response to inflammatory or immunological stimuli, may give rise to multiple polyps in the small and large intestine. The polyps can, however, be confined to the large intestine and then the condition may be confused with adenomatosis.

Finally, a further condition exists which also is not the classic form of polyposis coli. Unlike the two previous types, which are easily differentiated on histological examination, this is more difficult to separate, because it is both familial and adenomatous in character. The difference is mainly one of the mode of inheritance, being probably recessive instead of dominant as with polyposis coli. There is also a difference in degree as expressed in the number of adenomas present (see Chapter 9, "Differential Diagnosis").

With the exception of benign lymphoid polyposis, examples of each of the above three types of polyposis have been previously included in the adenomatosis material. They have now been removed and though not forming a large percentage of the total group, they did include proportionally more of the younger and older age groups. There has also been a great increase in the number of families available for study since they were written up by Dukes in 1952. Furthermore, an additional eighteen years of follow-up has been added to the earlier families, some of which have now been observed personally for over forty years.

The necessity of reviewing the histology of the tumors in cases of polyposis has led to a closer study of adenomas in polyposis coli and, in particular, to the earliest stages of their development.

For these reasons it has been considered necessary to assess the effect of these changes on previously published data and to review the clinical and histopathological aspects of adenomatous polyposis coli.

2

the st. mark's hospital
polyposis register

The present work is based on the records contained in the St. Mark's Hospital Polyposis Register. The Register was started in 1925 around a nucleus of three families reported by J. P. Lockhart-Mummery. Over the years, all forms of polyposis of the gastrointestinal tract have been included, and the Register now contains 294 families of which 200 are of the adenomatous type. Definitions of the terms used are as follows:

a) *Polyposis family*

A polyposis family is one in which at least one member suffers from multiple polyps of the gastrointestinal tract.

b) *Polyposis coli (adenomatous) family*

A family in which at least one member suffers from multiple polyps of the large intestine, the nature of the polyps having been diagnosed on histological grounds as adenomatous.

c) *"Polyposis coli patient"*

Group I. This group comprises those patients mentioned in the above definition of a polyposis family, i.e., one who has multiple intestinal polyps that have been proved to be adenomatous on histological evidence. This statement is not complete without some explanation of "multiple." "How many polyps make polyposis?" is an often asked question and, as will be shown in Chapter 9, there is now reason to believe that a numerical answer is available. The figure is in the region of 100 adenomas in the whole large intestine, most cases of adenomatosis being far in excess of this. The number of patients in this group where histological confirmation was available is 309.

If other family members, not conforming strictly to this definition, were discarded, a distorted picture of the disease would result, and much valuable information would be lost. For these reasons the following groups of patients are considered also to have suffered from polyposis on the basis of a high degree of probability.

Group II. Any parent, sibling, or child of a Group I patient known to have had polyps of unknown histology and cancer of the large intestine (71 cases).

Group III. Any parent, sibling or child of Group I patients known to have had cancer of the large intestine (184 cases).

These last two groups are made up largely from representatives of generations prior to that of the propositus and will be proportionately less as the families are followed up.

Group IV. Parents, siblings, or children of Group I patients who have polyps of unknown histology but no known evidence of bowel cancer (43 cases).

Group V. Individuals in whom there was no evidence of either intestinal cancer or of polyps, but whose parents or siblings had polyposis, and who transmitted the disease to their children. The explanation of such cases is either incomplete knowledge of the medical history or death before polyposis manifested itself (10 cases).

The total number of individuals in the 200 polyposis families considered under the above definitions to have had the disease is 617.

d) "Member of polyposis family"

Some few "families" in the Register consist of one person only, i.e., the propositus about whose relatives nothing could be learned. At the other extreme, the largest family contains 144 persons. Though it is necessary to record all ramifications of the family, not all the individuals recorded are at risk of inheriting the disease. Inheritance of polyposis is of the dominant type, where only 50% of the children are expected to develop adenomas. The unaffected children, though originally at risk, do not inherit polyposis and are normal in respect to the disease. Their children in turn are not at risk. From genetic considerations, therefore, the "members" of a polyposis family are defined as consisting of those individuals who have the disease, the brothers and sisters of affected persons, and the children of affected persons.

This definition may be too wide when applied to families with only one affected member, because if the patient is the result of a new mutation, his siblings are not at risk. It is not always possible to say whether such "solitary" cases are new mutations or merely appear so because of incomplete knowledge of the family, particularly when this is small.

The total number of persons recorded in the 200 families is 4,483, but the number of family members as defined above is 1,958, of which, as previously stated, 617 are considered to have had polyposis coli.

Of the 617 patients accepted for study, 170 were seen at St. Mark's

Hospital, the earliest being recorded in 1918. Of these 138 underwent major surgery in the hospital and, with the exception of a few of the earliest cases, detailed reports, photographs, and sections of the operation specimens were available for study. At least 31 colectomy specimens removed elsewhere from family members had been sent to the Pathology Department of St. Mark's Hospital for examination.

INVESTIGATION OF THE FAMILY

Investigation of a polyposis family usually begins when a patient presents with symptoms which are found clinically or radiologically to be due to multiple intestinal tumors. The patient, who is the propositus, is questioned about his children; his brothers and sisters and their children; his parents and their siblings, the family pedigree being traced backwards and laterally as far as possible. Names, especially maiden names of married women, addresses, dates of birth and death are obtained where possible. Further details are sought of causes of death, hospitals where treated, when, and by whom. Every statement is recorded, for however trivial it seems at the time, it may later prove to be a vital clue. Confirmation of medical histories is obtained from hospitals and other sources and a provisional family pedigree prepared. At this stage the pedigree usually contains a number of errors, some latent and others obvious, such as when, due to mistakes in dates and ages, it appears that a family member had three children before the age of 12 years. These are corrected by further interviews, either with the first informant or with other family members with better memories. Names which emerge are compared with those in the name index of the Register, now numbering over 1,200, in the hope of finding linkages with known families.

Efforts are now made to persuade as many family members as possible to be examined so that further latent disease may be discovered and treated. As will be shown, the disease rarely manifests itself before the age of 14 years, and it is at this time that periodic sigmoidoscopic examinations are started. An "Advanced Appointments" system is organized in yearly groups. Thus the details of a child at risk, aged 6 years in 1968, are entered on a card filed under 1976, which acts as a reminder that the child has then reached the age at which examinations should start. If sigmoidoscopy reveals no polyps, it is repeated in 2 to 3 years' time and the patient's card advanced the appropriate number of years in the file. At the moment there are 177 children under the age of 14 years awaiting follow-up. No definite age can be given beyond which examinations can be discontinued if persistently negative. It can only be stated that with increasing age the risk of developing polyposis falls rapidly.

The recording of the family history is a continuous process which must be pursued through successive generations. As with brandy, the family history increases in value with age, and it is fortunate that the Register contains some families that have been observed for more than forty years. Pedigrees of Family No. 1, made in 1925 and again in 1973, are reproduced in Figure 1 and give a graphic idea of the value of prolonged observation.

3

genetic and epidemiological features of familial polyposis coli

INHERITANCE

Following Cripps's first observation in 1882 of two siblings with polyposis coli, evidence has accumulated confirming the hereditary nature of the disease, culminating in the papers of Dukes (1952) and Veale (1965). It is now considered to be a dominant character carried on a single gene and affecting each generation. Apparent skips are possible (10 cases occur in the present series as defined in Group V of polyposis patients), but these are almost certainly the result of incomplete knowledge. The character is not sex-linked and can be passed by either sex to either sex indiscriminately. The ratio of the sexes should, therefore, be equal, and this is approximately so in this series (54.1% males and 45.9% females). Although the proportion of affected and unaffected children should be the same, affected persons appear to be fewer, probably due to the late appearance of the polyps in a proportion of the cases. Various estimates of the manifestation of the disease have been made (Dukes 1952; Duhamel et al. 1960; Veale 1965) and these have been in the region of 80%.

So far no means have been found of indicating which children of a polyposis parent will develop the disease. Genetic markers, such as blood groups, have been unsuccessfully sought (Veale 1958). By electron microscopy Birbeck and Dukes (1963) have found granules in the apical part of epithelial cells from the mucous membrane and adenomas of polyposis cases, but, though there was a high degree of correlation, these findings were not specific. Dukes even enlisted the aid of a Scotland Yard fingerprint expert in an attempt to predetermine the future sufferer from polyposis. Utsunomiya and Nakamura (1975) found an increased opacity of the jaw bone in the majority of polyposis patients examined radiologically, but the value of this observation as a preclinical indication of polyposis is not known. The only sure method is that now employed of sigmoidoscopy of all children in these families.

Solitary Cases ("nonfamilial polyposis")

Sometimes no history can be found of similar disease in the relatives of a polyposis patient. The patient has either inherited the disease, in which case medical knowledge of the family is incomplete, or has developed the disease as the result of a new mutation. In the absence of precise information about such solitary patients it is usually assumed that a new mutation is responsible. These individuals are often said to have "nonfamilial polyposis." Though strictly true, the term may mislead by implying an absence of genetic factor. It must be emphasized that the children of such a patient are just as much at risk of developing polyps as are the children of patients with strong family histories.

In 90 of the 200 families in this survey there is no history of any member other than the propositus having the disease. Originally there were 9 additional solitary case families but in 8 of these, children of the propositus subsequently developed polyposis, and in the ninth case another brother became affected some years later. Thus, since the inception of the Register, 98 families appear to have been initiated through possible new mutations, or almost one-half of the total number investigated. This is probably too high a proportion, and in some, at least, of the solitary cases the whole truth has not emerged. A more accurate estimate of the true incidence is likely to be in the region of one-third.

Comparison of the characteristics of the disease as observed in the solitary case and in the multiple history cases shows little difference. The average age, age distribution, number of polyps, and the incidence rate of associated malignancy are similar. A slight variation in the sex ratio of the solitary cases (males 62.2%, females 37.8%) could alter as more cases accumulate. The "nonfamilial" patient must be regarded as an example of genuine adenomatosis coli.

GEOGRAPHICAL DISTRIBUTION

It is not surprising that the majority of reports of polyposis coli have come from those countries with the more sophisticated medical services, such as Great Britain, the United States of America, and Northern European countries. The heaviest concentration of reported polyposis thus falls in areas inhabited by the Caucasian race.

However, the disease is known to occur in other races. The St. Mark's Hospital Register contains the records of four Arabs (two from Egypt and one each from Kuwait and Lebanon) and of three West Indian families. The disease was almost certainly present in another Jamaican negro seen at St. Mark's, but this case was excluded from the series for lack of histological confirmation. Occurrence in American negroes has been mentioned by Cole et al. (1961), Gordon et al. (1962), and Dunning and Ibrahim (1955), and in South African Bantu negroes (Bremner 1965; McQuade & Stewart 1972). The Far East has produced examples in Japan (Kodaira 1964; Nishimura et al. 1969; Tajima et al. 1973) and Korea (Kim & Kim 1966). Two Indian families are included in the St. Mark's Hospital series. It is probable that no race or nationality is exempt, and it seems likely that the incidence is fairly constant throughout the world.

INCIDENCE OF POLYPOSIS COLI IN THE GENERAL POPULATION

Several attempts have been made to solve the difficult problem of estimating the proportion of polyposis coli patients in the general population. Scarborough and Klein (1948) analyzed the records of 10,000 patients and found 458 with benign polypoid disease, 23 of whom had 20 or more polyps, an incidence of 1 in 435. It will be shown later that the number of polyps is important and that a figure of 20 is certainly too low to be acceptable as a case of polyposis coli. Neel (1954) used a crude, indirect method and arrived at a figure of 1 in 29,000. The following year Reed and Neel (1955) refined the technique and obtained a rate of 1 in 8,300, which they thought might well be an underestimate. Veale's investigation of the St. Mark's Hospital material gave a frequency of 1 in 23,790 (Veale 1965). On the other hand, a more recent estimate has been made on a large family investigated by Pierce (1968) who found a value of 1 in 6,850. Alm and Licznerski (1973), using the excellent population records in Sweden to collect 97 polyposis families, calculated the incidence there to be 1 in 7,646.

If the average annual number of births for England and Wales for the first sixty years of this century is taken to be about three-quarters of a million, and if the incidence of polyposis is about 1 in 24,000, the number of persons with polyposis born each year is just over 30. Scotland would probably add another 2 or 3 to this. Veale also calculated the manifestation of the disease to be about 80%, giving the number of patients likely to develop polyposis each year as about 25.

In the St. Mark's Hospital series, patients born from 1900 onward have been arranged in yearly cohorts. In the first 40 years (1900–39) there are 328 patients, or an average of about 8 per year. There were also about another 50 patients who were either known to have had adenomatous polyposis but whose year of birth was unknown, or who had what was almost certainly adenomatous polyposis for which there was no histological confirmation. These raise the annual total to about 9 patients. Some apparently unaffected family members born in this period may yet develop the disease, but these will not increase the total by much. The cases recorded in the St. Mark's Hospital Register may, therefore, represent about one-third of the total polyposis coli in the United Kingdom, if the estimate made by Veale is correct, and about one-tenth if the other estimates are more accurate. Unfortunately, there is no way at the moment of telling which is correct.

SEX INCIDENCE

The total of 617 patients in the series is made up of 334 males (54.1%) and 283 females (45.9%). In the cohort series between 1900 and 1939 there were 241 patients who had an affected parent and these included 130 males (53.9%) and 111 females (46.1%). During the same period 67 "solitary" patients (i.e., possible mutants) were also born, but with these the 43 males exceeded the 24 females almost in the ratio of 3 to 2 (64.2% and 35.8% respectively).

AGE INCIDENCE

It is not possible to use the whole 617 cases when investigating the age incidence of the disease. Normally this is based on the age at diagnosis, but in this series of polyposis patients three groups can be identified, each of which has its own special contribution to make toward further knowledge of the disease.

1. Propositus group

These patients came for advice because they had symptoms. From this source, numbering 293 persons, details of symptoms and their duration, age at diagnosis, and incidence of associated malignancy were obtained.

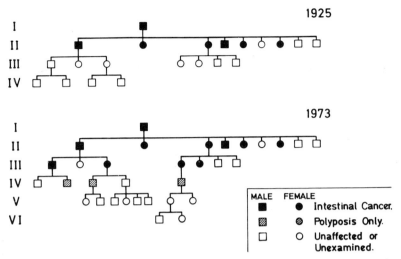

Fig. 1.   Pedigree of a polyposis family at the time of first contact and again 48 years later. In the interval four individuals in Generation III developed polyposis and cancer. Three other family members in Generation IV were affected, but because they were known to be at risk, colectomies were carried out before carcinoma supervened.

2. Call-up group

This comprises those relatives of patients known to have the disease and who, because of this, were called up for examination and found to be affected. Some of these patients had symptoms for which they had not sought advice, but most were symptomless. Obviously, this group, which numbered 117, were cases caught at an earlier stage than the propositus group.

3. Indeterminate group

In 207 patients little is known other than that they died from intestinal cancer and, in most cases, at what age. It is not generally known when or under what conditions they sought medical attention, though probably most would have been included in the propositus group if their full history were known. Apart from information useful to the genetic aspect of the disease, the main value of this group was in the calculation of the age at death from cancer.

In considering the age incidence of polyposis it seemed reasonable to base this on the age of the propositus group. In 12 patients the age was unknown, but analysis of the other 281 cases showed the average age at the time of diagnosis to be 36.3 years for males and 35.1 years for females. The age distribution is shown in Table 1 and illustrated in Figure 2, from which it will be seen that the curves rise fairly steeply to a peak in the region of 30 years and then decline more slowly to about 70 years.

The proportion of the total cases diagnosed at increasing age is demonstrated in Table 2, Figure 3. At 35 years of age only one-half of the group has been diagnosed, and at 50 years of age there were still more than 10% undiagnosed. This graph is useful in estimating the risk at various ages that apparently unaffected children of a polyposis parent may still develop the disease.

Environmental Factors

The role of a genetic factor in polyposis coli is now well established. If, as seems highly probable, most intestinal carcinomas develop from adenomas, the existence of a similar factor in respect of adenomatous tumors in the general population is also a possibility (Lovett 1974). It is conceivable that this genetic factor is modified by environmental influences either in the direction of intensifying or of neutralizing the adenoma-producing process. No environmental factors have been identified, but that they exist is very probable. The increase in cancer of the colon among Japanese immigrants to the United States of America who adopt a more westernized type of diet is possibly evidence of a variation in the incidence of the disease due to a change in external factors (Wynder et al. 1969; Haenszel & Kurihara 1968).

One of the factors could be increased contact with carcinogen substances such as are known to produce neoplastic tumors in the colon of rats (Laqueur 1965; Spjut & Noall 1971). As most intestinal cancers appear to arise from adenomas, it may be said that cancer is an end-product of some adenomas. If so, carcinogens may act by first producing benign epithelial tumors, some of which progress to cancer by an inevitable biological sequence; or it may be that this subsequent step has to be initiated by more intense or prolonged exposure to the carcinogen or by the further action of some other substance. It is significant that the administration to rats of 3-2' dimethyl-4-aminobiphenyl produces both adenomas as well as adenocarcinomas, and that some of the microscopic appearances seen in sections from the colons of affected rats closely resemble those seen in polyposis patients. Substances that are capable of producing or modifying neoplastic change might be ingested with food, or formed by the action of bacteria on either food or the digestive secretions, such as bile (Hill et al. 1971; Drasar & Hill 1972). In

Table 1. Age distribution of polyposis patients at time of diagnosis. Propositus group (293 cases)

Age in years	Males No.	Males %	Females No.	Females %	Total No.	Total %
0–	1	0.6	—	—	1	0.4
5–	—	—	—	—	—	—
10–	2	1.3	1	0.8	3	1.1
15–	8	5.1	4	3.2	12	4.3
20–	15	9.6	14	12.1	29	10.3
25–	24	15.3	26	20.2	50	17.8
30–	25	15.9	21	16.9	46	16.3
35–	24	15.3	22	17.7	46	16.3
40–	23	14.7	13	10.5	36	12.8
45–	16	10.2	12	9.7	28	10.0
50–	8	5.1	6	4.9	14	5.0
55–	6	3.8	3	2.4	9	3.2
60–	3	1.9	1	0.8	4	1.4
65–	1	0.6	—	—	1	0.4
70–	1	0.6	1	0.8	2	0.7
Not stated	9		3		12	
TOTAL	166	100.0	127	100.0	293	100.0
Average age:	36.3 yrs		35.1 yrs		35.8 yrs	

Table 2. Relationship of age and percentage of total cases of polyposis diagnosed (281 propositus cases)

Age group	No. of cases diagnosed	Percentage of total cases
0–5	1	0.4
0–10	1	0.4
0–15	4	1.4
0–20	16	5.7
0–25	46	16.4
0–30	96	34.2
0–35	142	50.5
0–40	188	66.9
0–45	223	79.4
0–50	251	89.3
0–55	265	94.3
0–60	274	97.5
0–65	278	98.9
0–70	279	99.3
0–75	281	100.0

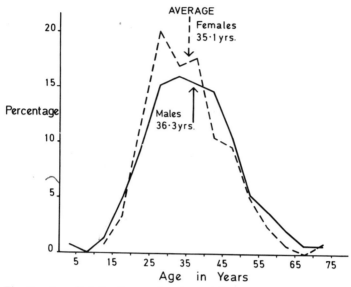

Fig. 2. Age distribution at the time of diagnosis of males and females with polyposis (281 propositus cases).

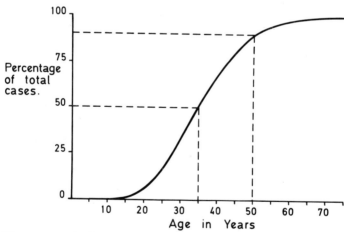

281 PROPOSITUS CASES

Fig. 3. Graph showing the percentage of polyposis cases diagnosed at different ages. At 35 years of age half the cases have been diagnosed, but at 50 years there are still more than 10% of the propositus patients who have not yet presented.

this connection the effect of diet on bowel motility could be important (Birkett 1971).

Nullification of the genetic factor by environmental influences is indicated by the regression and disappearance of rectal polyps in some patients when colectomy and ileorectal anastomosis has been carried out for polyposis. What this inhibiting factor might be is quite unknown, although a chemical substance in the ileal contents, change in blood supply, or an increase in the effectiveness of host resistance when most of the diseased bowel has been removed have all been suggested (Cole & Holden 1959). The effect is, however, of a limited nature, and in most cases the adenomas reappear after varying periods of time.

The relationship of genetic and environmental factors in the production of neoplasms is a complex problem for the solution of which little information is available. The nature of these factors and their mode of interaction is practically unknown. It is possible that all epithelial cells of the large intestine in all individuals are capable of neoplastic change, and that in familial polyposis coli the genetic factor is an inherited ability to produce a carcinogen. This, however, implies that the process of adenoma formation is totally inherited, which is contrary to experience. It could be that a defect is inherited, which although insufficient in itself to produce adenomas, can do so when an additional factor is introduced from the environment. This would have to be ubiquitous, otherwise polyposis would not manifest itself so clearly as a Mendelian dominant. Alternatively, the inherited character may be an inability to produce a factor inhibitory to adenoma formation. It is possible that several factors are necessary and that in polyposis all or most of these are inherited, making the advent of adenomas a relatively self-contained and automatic process, subject only to limited modification by noninherited conditions.

The regression of rectal polyps after colectomy could result from the introduction of a further factor that interrupts the sequence of necessary steps in tumor formation or maintenance. With the recessive type of adenomatosis the inherited factors would appear to act in a far less intense and widespread fashion than in polyposis coli. This might mean that fewer of the factors are inherited and more have to be acquired. It is obvious that a great deal more needs to be known before any reliable solutions to these problems can be given. In our present state of ignorance it is possible only to say that the available evidence suggests that genetic and environmental factors are involved, but that the nature and relative importance of these has yet to be determined.

4
pathology of familial polyposis coli

a) GENERAL PATHOLOGY

Familial polyposis coli is an hereditary disease in which the large intestine contains numerous tumors composed of neoplastic epithelium arising from the mucous membrane (Fig. 4). Three benign types of such tumors are usually recognized (Morson 1968).

1) Tubular adenoma. This is the most common type of benign neoplastic tumor arising from the mucus-secreting epithelium lining the interior of the intestine. The epithelial glands differ from normal tubules in that they are lined by cells having hyperchromatic nuclei, increased mitotic activity, and decreased mucus production, and that the cells are stratified, being arranged in multiple layers (Figs. 5 & 6). Macroscopically adenomatous tumors are lobulated growths, irregularly spheroid or oval in shape, seldom more than 3 cms in diameter, and usually attached by long stalks to the bowel wall (Fig. 7), though occasionally they may be sessile and up to 10 cms in diameter.

2) Villous adenoma. These are epithelial tumors of similar histology to that of adenomas as far as the cells are concerned, but these now line delicate strands of connective tissue, forming long villi with little branching, the tips of which are usually pointed (Fig. 8). Mucus production is generally much more in evidence than in the tubular adenomas. The gross appearances, however, differ greatly from those of adenomas, as villous adenomas are mainly sessile growths covering large areas of bowel, sometimes measuring up to 12 or 15 cms in the longest axis. The surface is shaggy or villous in appearance (Fig. 9).

3) Tubulo-villous (papillary) adenoma. The two tumors described above under the terms "tubular adenoma" and "villous adenoma" are not distinct histological types, but represent the two extremes of a range of epithelial tumors that fade imperceptibly into each other. In between, there is a group in which the histology is intermediate, between tubular and villous; for these tumors the term "tubulo-villous" is convenient, although "papillary adenoma" has also been used. Histologically these tumors differ from tubular adenomas in that they form villi, but these are shorter and more branched than those seen in villous adenomas and have blunt or rounded ends. Sometimes tumors are a mixture of tubular and villous forms, and these are also included in this group.

The smooth graduation between all these types of tumors suggests that they are only minor variants of what is essentially the same tendency to neoplastic overgrowth of the intestinal mucosa. It is possible that the differences may relate to the stroma formation rather than to epithelial activity. The term "adenoma" is used subsequently to describe all forms of benign neoplastic epithelial hyperplasia. The majority of the tumors found in familial polyposis are tubular adenomas (adenomatous polyps).

b) MACROSCOPIC PATHOLOGY

1. Number of Polyps

Familial polyposis coli is also called "multiple polyposis" or "multiple adenomatosis," but it has not been considered necessary to define "multiple" in this connection. It obviously means more than one, but in some reports it has meant very few in addition.

In the period 1965 to 1969, eighteen colectomy specimens removed for polyposis were received for examination in the Pathology Department of St. Mark's Hospital. With each of these considerable care was taken to ascertain as accurately as possible the number of polyps present (Fig. 10). Two difficulties were encountered in the actual counting. The polyps are generally gradated in size and it was not easy to decide when a polyp was too small to count. The tumor had to be visible to the naked eye and palpable as a projection above the mucosa when a probe was gently drawn over it. These lower limit growths are around 1.5 mms in diameter and their macroscopic and microscopic appearances are shown in Figures 11 and 12. The other difficulty experienced was that in a few specimens the tumors were so sessile and numerous as to appear confluent (Figs. 13 & 14).

The total number of polyps per specimen varied from 157 to 3,676, and the average was 981. Reasonably accurate estimates had been made in 9 other specimens removed prior to 1965, and to these have been added those of another 30 colons received since 1969. In this group of 39 cases the range was from 104 to over 5,000 adenomas,

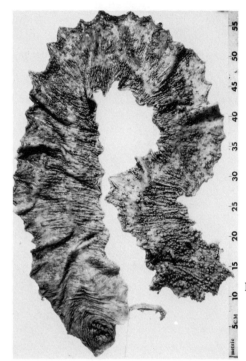

Fig. 4. Total colectomy specimen which has been opened up and pinned out before fixation to demonstrate the polyps to the best advantage.

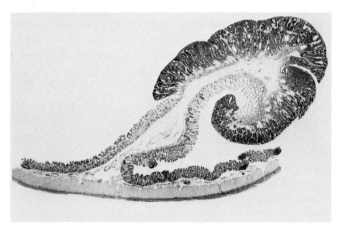

Fig. 5. Pedunculated adenoma of the rectum. The stalk is formed by an extension of the normal mucosa and is in sharp contrast with the hyperchromatic adenomatous overgrowth of the tumor. (×7) (Reduced by 30%)

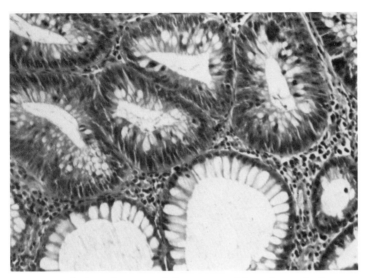

Fig. 6. Tubular adenoma of the rectum. There is marked hyperchromatism, stratification of the epithelial cells, and loss of mucus secretion. (×290) (Reduced by 35%)

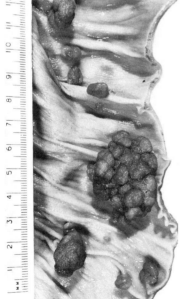

Fig. 7. Portion of colon removed for polyposis. The largest tumor present shows the characteristic lobulated surface of an adenoma.

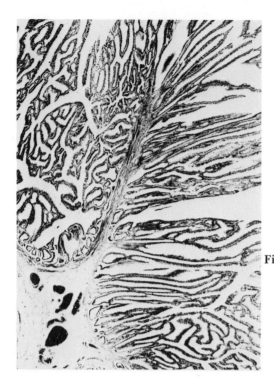

Fig. 8. Villous adenoma from a case of polyposis. The tumor is composed of long fronds consisting of a delicate stroma covered by a layer of neoplastic epithelial cells, most of which are actively secreting mucus. (×7) (Reduced by 40%)

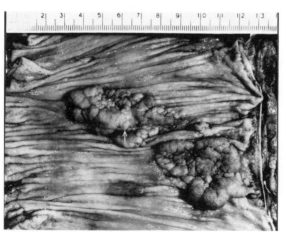

Fig. 9. Two sessile tumors of the transverse colon from a polyposis patient. Microscopic examination showed these to be mainly villous adenomas. The arrow indicates an area of superficial ulceration and induration which proved to be a small focus of invasive adenocarcinoma.

Table 3. Distribution of cases according to the number of polyps present in the large intestine

Number of polyps	Specially counted cases	Cases with approximate counts	Based on photographs	Total
0–100	—	—	—	—
100–200	1	2	11	14
200–500	4	13	22	39
500–1000	9	10	25	44
1000+	4	14	10	28
TOTAL	18	39	68	125

with an average of just over 1,000. Since 1933 photographs of operation specimens have been attached routinely to the pathology reports, and though it was not possible from these to give an accurate polyp count, it was relatively easy to state a minimal number, which was certainly an underestimate of the actual number of polyps present. Estimates were made in 68 such cases. Table 3 shows the numerical distribution of these three groups of cases. It will be seen that in no specimen was there less than 100 polyps and only 14 had less than 200. Since in 11 of these, the figure is almost certainly an underestimate, it may be said that few cases of polyposis coli have less than 200 polyps. For practical purposes, therefore, "multiple" adenomatosis may be defined as a condition where 100 or more adenomas are present in the large intestine. The diagnostic significance of this figure will be discussed in regard to "recessive" polyposis (see Chapter 9, "Differential diagnosis").

2. Density of Polyps

In the series of eighteen colectomy specimens where the tumors were counted, an estimate was made of the surface area of the mucosa of the fixed specimen from its length and average width. The total mucosal surface of the whole colectomy specimen was found to be generally between 700 and 1,400 sq cms, with an average of just over 1,000 sq cms. As the number of polyps was known, the density could be calculated. This was found to vary from 0.15 to 3.0 polyps per sq cm. The lower figure was exceptional, and a second definition of polyposis may be made on the basis of density, that it is a disease where there is at least one polyp present on each 5 sq cms of mucosal surface. Examples of low and high polyp density are shown in Figures 15 and 16. The close proximity of the adenomas when

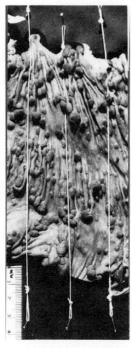

Fig. 10. Method used to count the polyps. The mucosal surface is divided into narrow strips by threads. The two areas shown each contain about 50 tumors.

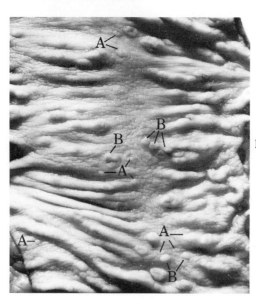

Fig. 11. Photograph of the mucosal surface showing numerous small polyps and sessile nodules. The smaller tumors (marked "A"), though almost certainly adenomatous in nature, were ignored in the counting. Those marked "B" represent the lower limit of size considered worthy of inclusion as polyps.

24 **FAMILIAL POLYPOSIS COLI**

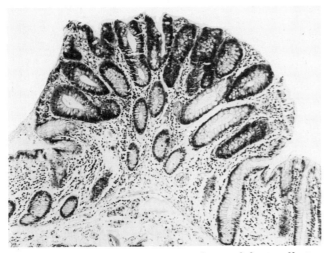

Fig. 12. Microscopic appearance of one of the smallest tumors counted. About ten tubules are involved in the adenomatous proliferation. (×100) (Reduced by 40%)

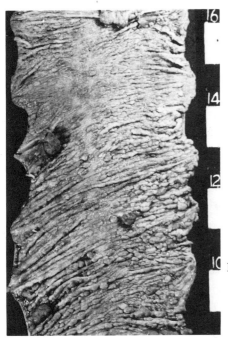

Fig. 13. Surface appearance of the mucosa in a colectomy specimen removed for polyposis. Some definite polyps are present but most of the surface is covered by confluent sessile tumors.

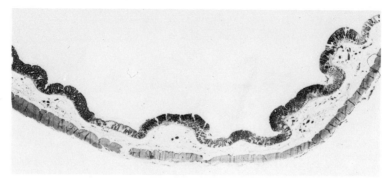

Fig. 14. Low power view of the mucosa from an area of confluent tumors, showing sessile patches of adenomatous proliferation separated by narrow zones of apparently normal mucous membrane. (×7) (Reduced by 30%)

present in high density is shown in a low power microphotograph in Figure 17.

3. Distribution of Polyps

Before discussing the distribution of adenomas around the colon it should be said that the polyps are confined to the large intestine and do not involve the small intestine. A few instances are known where adenomas, usually solitary, have been found in the small bowel. These are described in Chapter 6, "Associated lesions," and may be coincidental findings. The terminal ileum may contain polypoid tumors which are claimed to be adenomatosis extending into the small bowel (Fig. 18), but if these ileal tumors are examined microscopically, they are found to be hyperplastic lymphoid follicles (Fig. 19).

The appendix as part of the large intestine shares its liability to adenomatous overgrowth. Sections through the appendix often show definite adenomatous proliferation either within the mucosa (Fig. 20) or less commonly as small polyps (Fig. 21).

The total number of polyps has been discussed in the previous section, but not the distribution of these polyps around the colon. Information on this point was collected from the eighteen colectomy specimens in which the polyps were counted. The counting had been carried out in three stages:

1. Right colon, i.e., from ileocecal valve to hepatic flexure.
2. Transverse colon, from hepatic flexure to the splenic flexure.

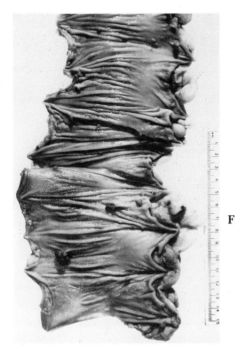

Fig. 15. Portion of colectomy specimen removed for polyposis. Relatively few polyps are present, the whole specimen containing only 480 with an overall density of 0.35 per sq. cm. The tumors were less numerous in the sigmoid segment illustrated above, the density being about 0.2 tumors per sq. cm.

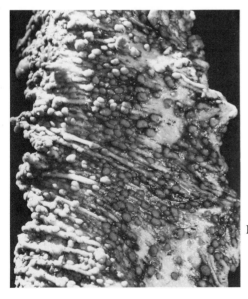

Fig. 16. Close-up photograph of a colon with dense polyp population, 3 tumors per sq. cm. or 3,676 tumors in the colectomy specimen.

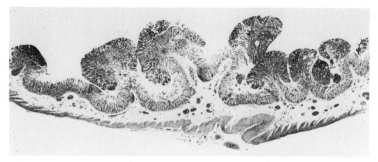

Fig. 17. Section from a colon with high density polyposis. In a strip of colon wall little more than two centimeters in length there are at least nine adenomas. (×7) (Reduced by 30%)

3. Left colon, from the splenic flexure to the distal end of the specimen.

The approximate positions of the flexures on the fixed and open intestine were identified as the proximal and distal points of attachment of the greater omentum. The rectum was removed in only two of the eighteen specimens. The counts for the three segments of the colon are given in Table 4. On average number alone the tendency is for the polyps to increase in number from the proximal to the distal end and supports the general impression that the polyps are more common on the left side of the colon than on the right. On the other hand, a comparison of the average densities shows that, as before, the polyps were densest in the left colon (1.07 per sq cm); the density in the transverse colon was less than in the right colon (0.83 per sq cm and 0.95 per sq cm respectively). This probably indicates a greater surface area in the transverse segment. However, both methods of comparison, number and density, agree on the highest incidence of polyps on the right side in five cases, the transverse two cases only, and the left colon in eleven instances.

Further information about distribution was obtained from 68 reports in which comparative densities in the three regions were mentioned. In 17 specimens the distribution was said to be uniform; in 16 the polyps increased from cecum to sigmoid, and in only one case were there more polyps in the right colon than the left. The remaining 34 specimens showed a more patchy distribution of tumors, the right colon being mentioned as the area of most polyps in 5 cases, the transverse colon in 3, the left colon in 13 with the remaining 13 cases indefinite. It was not possible to give figures for the number and density of polyps in the rectum, which was seldom removed. If removed, it was because it contained a carcinoma, and this might occupy a large proportion of the surface area and invalidate the count. On the evidence available, it is probable that conditions in the rectum are similar to those in the pelvic colon. In 2 reports there was a remark to the effect that the polyps were less numerous in the rectum than in the colon, but in none of the 170 patients seen at St. Mark's Hospital has the rectum ever been completely free from polyps, although in one there were only a few adenomas.

Occasionally an unusual distribution pattern is seen, as for instance when there are few polyps in the right colon but a heavy concentration from the hepatic flexure to the rectum (Fig. 22). This curious distribution, present in all five affected members of a sibship (none of whom was more than 18 years of age at the time of colectomy), appears to be a family characteristic.

4. Size of Polyps

Considerable differences exist in the size of the adenomatous tumors present in the intestine in polyposis. In order to obtain more information on this point, not only were the polyps counted in the eighteen colectomy specimens previously mentioned, but an attempt was made to estimate the size distribution. The method used was to measure the diameter of sample polyps and roughly to gauge the proportion below 0.5 cms in diameter and between 0.5 cms and 1.0 cms. Tumors above 1 cm in size were individually measured and counted. Polyp size is related to the degree of maturity of the disease and to the time at which the natural course of the disease was interrupted by surgery. This is reflected in Table 5, which gives the approximate numbers and proportions of polyps of different sizes found in 13 late (propositus) cases and 15 early (call-up) cases. Polyps over 0.5 cms in diameter constitute 11% of all tumors in the late cases, as against 2% in the early cases. What is of more interest perhaps is the fact that only 1% of all tumors, even in the late cases, are over 1 cm in diameter. This is the size that has significance for clinicians as being that at which the malignant potential of the adenoma may begin to manifest itself (Grinnell & Lane 1958; Welin et al. 1963; Scarborough 1965). The largest benign tumor in this series was a sessile adenoma measuring 5.0 cms by 4.0 cms. Seven carcinomas were also present, three of which were larger than this, and, in general, cancers when present tended to be the largest tumors in the specimen, partly because of their greater growth rate

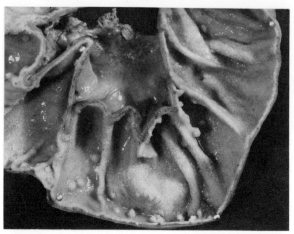

Fig. 18. Terminal ileum from a case of adenomatous polyposis coli, showing small polypoid lymphoid follicles sometimes thought to be an extension of the polyposis into the small intestine.

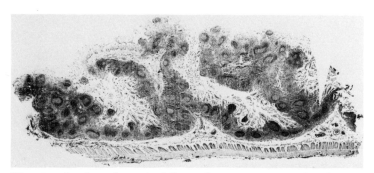

Fig. 19. Section of terminal ileum from a patient with polyposis coli. Hyperplasia of the lymphoid follicles has produced polypoid tumors. (×9) (Reduced by 30%)

and partly because the bigger polyps are more likely to undergo malignant degeneration.

In some specimens the polyps were of remarkably even size (Fig. 23), but in most there is considerable variation, though seldom as great as that shown in Figure 24, where nearly all the tumors are less than 0.5 cms in diameter, but one measures 3.7 cms across. It is not known whether such a tumor develops as a solitary polyp long before its fellows (which seems more probable) or has a particularly rapid growth rate. Such disparity, however, emphasizes the necessity of barium enema examination of the colon before deciding to postpone surgery in what appears to be an early case.

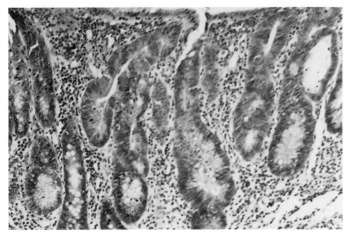

Fig. 20. Small area of dysplastic epithelium showing considerable atypia, found on routine examination of the appendix from a polyposis patient. (×160) (Reduced by 40%)

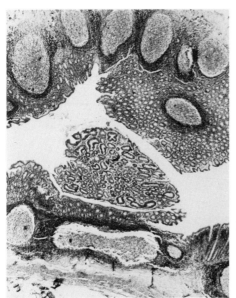

Fig. 21. Part of a longitudinal section through the appendix from a patient with polyposis, showing a small adenomatous polyp within the lumen. (×22) (Reduced by 40%)

5. Types of Polyps

The various forms which benign neoplastic growth of intestinal mucosa can assume have been described in the introduction to this section. At the two extremes there are the solid, lobulated, pedunculated, tubular adenomas and the shaggy, broad-based, villous adeno-

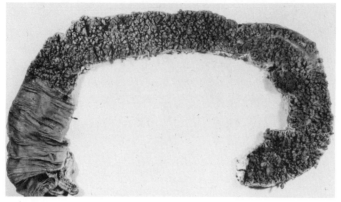

Fig. 22. Colectomy specimen showing a heavy concentration of polyps from the hepatic flexure to the sigmoid colon, but only a few are present in the ascending colon.

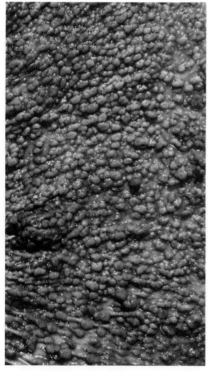

Fig. 23. Close-up photograph of a colectomy specimen in which more than 5,000 adenomatous tumors were present. Throughout the colon there was remarkably little variation in the size of the polyps.

Table 4. Relative distribution of polyps in the colon (18 cases)

	Average number of polyps	Average density of polyps (per sq cm)
Right colon	277	0.95
Transverse colon	312	0.83
Left colon	387	1.07

Table 5. Proportion of polyps of different sizes in early and late cases

Size of polyp	Propositus patients (13 cases)		Call-up patients (15 cases)	
	Number	Approximate proportion (%)	Number	Approximate proportion (%)
Less than 0.5 cm	12,650	89	8,440	98
0.5–1.0 cm	1,399	10	165	1.9
1.0–2.0 cms	130	1	7	0.08
Over 2.0 cms	8	< 0.1	1	0.01

mas. Between is a gradated series of intermediate forms. All these types can be found in polyposis coli as well as in the nonpolyposis tumors, though whether or not in the same proportions is not known, as no quantitative comparison is available. It is certainly difficult to find examples of villous adenomas in polyposis, and it is likely that papillary adenomas are not so common as among the nonpolyposis adenomas. Large adenomas are more likely to be found among the nonpolyposis tumors. These differences may, however, be a reflection of the number of tumors present. A solitary growth may have to acquire a considerable size before giving rise to symptoms, whereas the hundreds of adenomas in polyposis may produce similar symptoms when the tumors are still small and before they have had a chance to develop into different types. Age may be another factor influencing the type of polyp. The average age of nonpolyposis patients with villous tumors is about four years older than those with tubular adenomas.

c) MICROSCOPIC PATHOLOGY

1. General Histopathology of Polyps

The polyps present in polyposis coli are adenomatous polyps, i.e., neoplastic tumors consisting of an overgrowth of hyperplastic mucus-secreting intestinal epithelium supported on a stroma com-

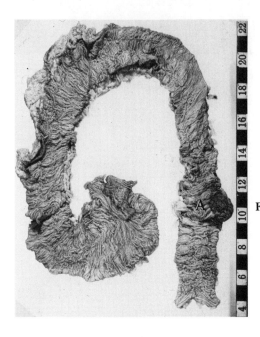

Fig. 24. Many small adenomatous polyps were present in this specimen, only a few of which can be discerned in the photograph. One exceptionally large adenoma is, however, situated in the upper sigmoid colon (A).

posed of loose connective tissue and blood vessels. According to the relative disposition of stroma and epithelial covering, different types of tumors are recognized by their macroscopic and microscopic appearances as tubular adenomas, villous adenomas, or the intermediate tubulo-villous adenomas, these having already been described in the previous section. As stated there, the term "adenoma" is used to cover all varieties of benign neoplastic epithelial tumors of the large intestine.

The tumors occurring in polyposis coli are, with rare exception, adenomas. Metaplastic polyps have been found in seven patients (Fig. 25). This tumor, described in Chapter 9, "Differential diagnosis," is so common that its coincidental association with polyposis coli is not surprising. The only other nonadenomatous tumor encountered in 140 colectomy specimens removed for polyposis has been a single example of a juvenile polyp or mucous retention polyp (see Chapter 9, "Differential diagnosis"). The presence of this tumor may have been coincidental, but could have been related to the polyposis coli, as there is a suspected genetic relationship which is discussed in Chapter 6, "Associated lesions."

2. Earliest stages of adenoma formation

The earliest stages in the development of intestinal adenomas have been little studied in patients with solitary or few tumors,

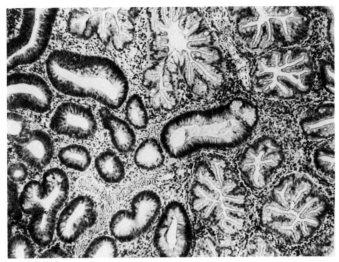

Fig. 25. Unusual juxtaposition of adenomatous tissue (*left*) and metaplastic epithelium (*right*) in a polyp. (×130) (Reduced by 35%)

because these growths are usually well advanced when discovered. Polyposis coli, however, is a condition that provides a unique opportunity for studying adenoma formation. Not only are hundreds of tumors of all sizes available for study, but between the visible polyps there are, in most cases, areas of microscopic hyperplasia from which other adenomas arise. The earliest changes detected in this epithelial hyperplasia are the same as those seen in mature adenomas, i.e., hyperchromatism, stratification of the epithelial cells, decreased mucus production, and increased mitotic activity. The main difference is the more limited area of involvement, which may often be a single tubule or crypt of Lieberkühn, such as is shown in vertical section in Figure 26 or in cross section in Figure 27. The hyperplasia may not involve the entire surface of the tubule, as can be seen in Figure 28, where only three-quarters of the circumference of the tubule has undergone neoplastic hyperplasia. This may be due to the section passing through a serrated junction of normal and hyperplastic epithelium. Rarely the abnormal epithelium can be seen budding off like a small diverticulum from the main glandular space, which is lined by a single layer of normal mucus-secreting cells (Fig. 29). The transition from normal to abnormal epithelium is not always easily found in sections, but when present is seen to be an abrupt process. Normally it is best seen in vertical sections of the colonic or rectal mucosa, when it is found about half way up the

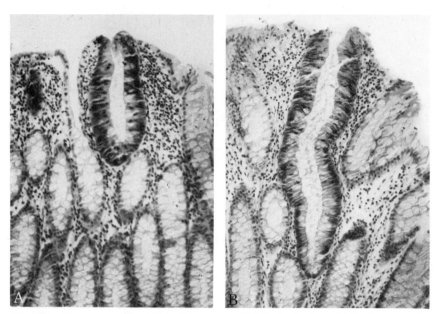

Fig. 26. Two examples of single crypts of Lieberkühn in which the normal mucus secreting cells lining the tubules have been replaced by hyperplastic epithelium similar to that found in adenomas. (×180) (Reduced by 40%)

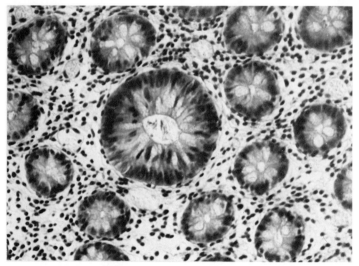

Fig. 27. Transverse section through the mucosa of a colon affected by polyposis coli. One tubule is lined by abnormal epithelium of the type found in adenomas and represents one of the earliest stages in the formation of the polyps.

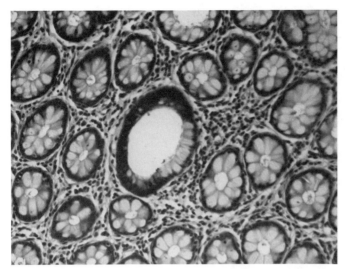

Fig. 28. Transverse section of mucosa showing one tubule with adenomatous changes which do not involve the entire circumference of the wall. (×225) (Reduced by 35%)

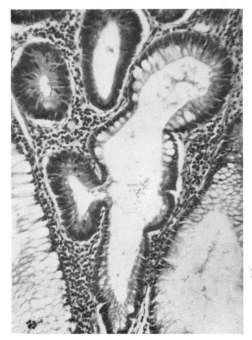

Fig. 29. Small duct lined with adenomatous epithelium budding off from a normal tubule. (×200) (Reduced by 40%)

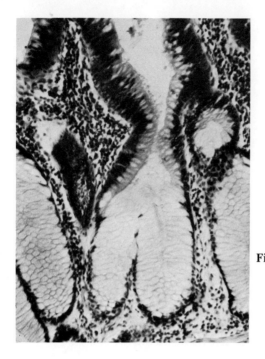

Fig. 30. Crypt of Lieberkühn showing normal epithelium in the lower half and adenomatous proliferation of the mucus secreting cells in the upper part. (×180) (Reduced by 40%)

crypts of Lieberkühn, which are undergoing hyperplasia (Fig. 30). This position has significance when related to the work of Cole and McKalen (1963) on the morphogenesis of adenomatous polyps in the human colon. Using tritiated thymidine in a patient about to undergo colectomy for polyposis, they found that though in the majority of sections taken through the mucosa the labeled cells were in the expected positions at the base of the crypts of Lieberkühn, in other cases the take-up of the thymidine occurred in the upper half of the crypts, suggesting some abnormal process of cellular replacement. This is the reverse of the conclusions drawn by Lane and Lev (1963) in their observations on the origin of adenomatous epithelium in the colon.

The study of these early adenomatous changes was facilitated by scanning as much mucosa as possible. One method of achieving this was by embedding flat portions of intestine mucosal-surface downward and cutting transverse serial sections through the mucous membrane. It was seldom that a section was obtained of the whole area of mucosa taken for examination, but in most cases adequate areas for study were present in at least some of the serial sections (Fig. 31). Although the area of mucosa was usually selected because it appeared to be free from adenomas, it will be seen that the regular

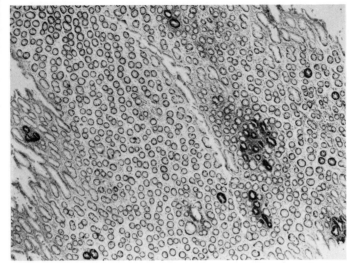

Fig. 31. Transverse section through apparently normal
mucosa from a colectomy specimen removed for
polyposis. A number of hyperchromatic hyperplastic
tubules are present, sometimes singly, sometimes in small
groups of two or three. The cluster of about eight abnormal
crypts toward the right of the picture probably represents
the base of an early adenoma only just visible to the naked
eye. (×18) (Reduced by 35%)

network of normal transverse tubules is splattered with crypts lined
by hyperplastic epithelium of the type seen in adenomas. Of the
specimens examined by this method, that illustrated above showed
the largest incidence of abnormal tubules, approximately one in one
hundred of the total crypts present. Where the affected tubules are
bunched into small groups, it is possible that each group represents
only one incipient adenoma. Even so, the number of possible further
adenomas illustrated in Figure 31 is about ten in an area of 0.5 sq
cms. This section was taken from the specimen that had most polyps
(3,676) among the cases in which comparisons were made, and it
would appear that there is a direct relationship between the number
of abnormal tubules and the density of adenomas present.

Similar studies of the mucosa in two cases of carcinoma of the
rectum without polyposis, as well as a review of sections of many
other intestinal cancer specimens, have not shown any similar
changes in the mucosa. Transverse mucosal sections were also taken
from a specimen containing twenty-eight adenomas, including two
which were malignant, and in these sections there was only one
group of tubules that might be considered to be hyperplastic. If

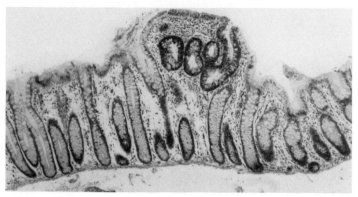

Fig. 32. Small area of adenomatous proliferation still contained mainly within the mucosa but commencing to produce a slight convexity of the mucosal surface. (×70) (Reduced by 40%)

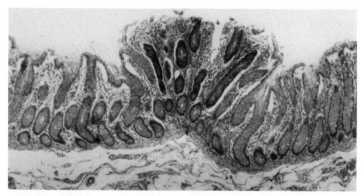

Fig. 33. Small group of hyperplastic tubules sprouting upward to project above the mucosal surface to form a tiny nodule invisible to the unaided eye. (×70) (Reduced by 40%)

adenomatous neoplasia is a common basis of both recessive and multiple adenomatosis, the relatively small number of polyps found in the former as compared with the latter may be a reflection of the relative frequency of hyperplastic tubules in the apparently normal mucosa in the two conditions.

3. Mode of formation of adenomas

The neoplastic changes seen in the single tubule may extend laterally to neighboring tubules, or these may undergo similar changes, giving rise to a slightly domed adenomatous proliferation

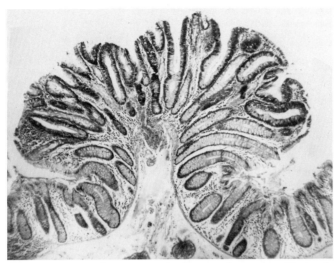

Fig. 34. Intermediate stage of adenoma formation. Upward extension of the tubules by adenomatous proliferation is forming a small tumor, traction on which has produced a stalk into which the muscularis mucosae is being drawn. (×70) (Reduced by 35%)

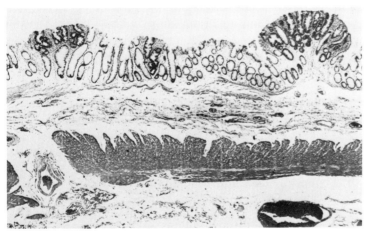

Fig. 35. Three stages of adenoma formation. In the center two hyperplastic tubules have produced slight doming of the mucosa. On the left there is a sessile elevation composed of about eight affected tubules, while at the right twice this number have formed a small adenoma. (×28) (Reduced by 30%)

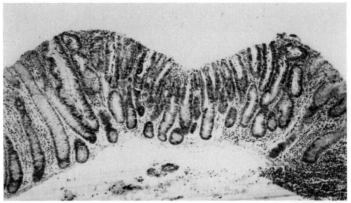

Fig. 36. Intramucosal hyperplasia taking the unusual form of a slight concavity in the mucosa. The glandular irregularity and the degree of dysplasia present are more than is ordinarily seen in such small lesions. (×70) (Reduced by 40%)

contained mainly within the thickness of the mucosa (Fig. 32), or it may be chiefly in an upward direction sprouting above the mucosal surface (Fig. 33). The latter, which is generally about 1 mm in diameter, is more frequently seen and probably represents the commonest origin of the pedunculated adenoma. Extension and branching of the neoplastic tubules soon produces a small polypoid lesion recognizable microscopically as a definite adenoma (Fig. 34). At this stage the tumor is about 3 mms in diameter and raised about 3 mms above the mucosal surface. From this point the adenoma enlarges and begins to exhibit those characteristics that will result in the tumor being classified as a tubular, villous or intermediate type of adenoma. The early stages of tumor formation can be found in close proximity to one another in polyposis specimens (Fig. 35).

The intramucosal lesions also usually proceed to polyp formation. More rarely, the intramucosal hyperplasia may take the form of a concave depression (Fig. 36). In this particular case the neoplastic tissue appears less differentiated than usual, and it is possible that such lesions undergo malignant degeneration more rapidly than do the polypoid forms and with less evidence of a benign origin. Such tumors could well be the forerunners of the tiny cancerous ulcers occasionally seen and may represent the nearest approach to what has been described as "de novo" cancer. However, these small malignant ulcers are exceedingly rare, and even with them a case can still be made for an origin in adenomatous tissue that is severely dysplastic from its beginning and that rapidly undergoes malignant degeneration.

Why in some instances comparatively few hyperplastic crypts are sufficient to give rise to small but definite tumors (Fig. 35), whereas more extensive neoplastic changes are confined still within the normal thickness of the mucosa (Fig. 37) is not known.

Another type of adenomatous proliferation takes the form of involvement of the upper part of the mucosa over a wide area (Fig. 38). Though less common than polyp formation it may occasionally be the predominant type of hyperplasia present, giving rise to confluent tumors similar to those seen in Figures 13 and 14. This superficial proliferation of the mucosa sometimes shows considerable hyperchromatism of the cells, with greatly reduced mucus production, and has been occasionally referred to as "surface cancer," although there is no evidence of invasion. These tumors usually develop into broad-based sessile adenomas, but if mucus production is maintained and villi are formed, the resulting tumor is the less commonly found villous adenoma. Figure 39 shows an example of this superficial hyperplasia proceeding to villous formation. Dukes (1947) probably had this type of tumor in mind when he suggested that villous papillomas and adenomas owed their differences to the site of origin of the hyperplasia within the crypts of Lieberkühn. The more recent work by Cole and McKalen mentioned above indicated, however, that this is not the correct explanation of the difference.

4. Comparison of Adenomas in Polyposis Patients and the General Population

As with the macroscopic characters, the histological appearances of benign epithelial tumors of the intestine, as found among non-polyposis patients, can be matched among the tumors occurring in the large intestine of polyposis coli patients. The tubular, villous and intermediate types of adenoma are all represented, though the villous tumor is less commonly encountered in polyposis patients.

Other features present in adenomatous tumors have also been compared. Gibbs (1967) has investigated the presence of argentaffin cells and Paneth cells in tubular and villous adenomas, from both nonpolyposis and polyposis cases, and found the incidence and density of these cells to be approximately the same for each.

In 1954 Leuchtenberger observed the frequent occurrence of inclusion bodies within the cytoplasm of benign and malignant tumors of the colon, and two years later reported, with his co-workers, the

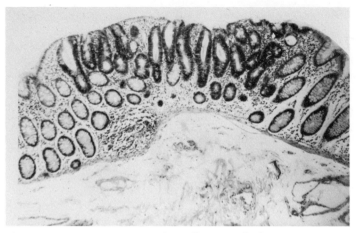

Fig. 37. Lesion consisting of a collection of adenomatous tubules, which have not produced any thickening of the mucosa. (×100) (Reduced by 40%)

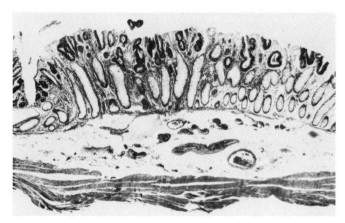

Fig. 38. Area of adenomatous proliferation confined to the upper layer of the mucosa, the lower part being normal. The hyperplastic tissue shows marked hyperchromatism with loss of mucus secretion and has sometimes been called, incorrectly, "surface cancer." (×45) (Reduced by 40%)

presence of similar bodies in the adenomas of polyposis coli. The bodies were thought to be viral in nature and possibly responsible for the production of intestinal tumors. However, subsequent electron microscopy investigations (Fisher & Sharkey 1962; Walb & Sandritter 1964) have shown that the bodies are inter- and not intra-

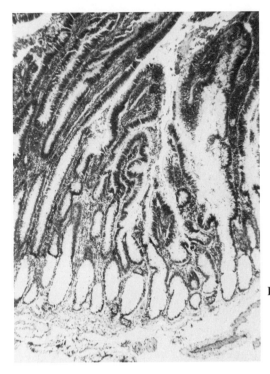

Fig. 39. Adenomatous hyperplasia arising from the upper part of the crypts of Lieberkühn and forming long villous projections. (×70) (Reduced by 40%)

cellular and do not have an internal structure resembling that of viruses. It is now considered that the particles are almost certainly nucleic debris from the breakdown of lymphocytes.

Of more interest are the ultramicroscopic granules described by Birbeck and Dukes (1963). In the course of electron microscopy of material from various intestinal lesions unusual granules were noticed in the epithelial cells of adenomas from a case of polyposis coli. These were present in varying numbers in most of the epithelial cells and were situated in the apical part of the cells just beneath the brush border. Further investigation showed similar granules in the epithelial cells of apparently unaffected areas of mucosa, between the polyps in polyposis specimens, and also in malignant cells in a cancer associated with polyposis. Altogether Birbeck and Dukes observed the granules in eleven of fourteen biopsies from polyposis specimens, while on the other hand twenty biopsies from non-polyposis cases were all negative. The particles were unlike Leuchtenberger's inclusion bodies, being much smaller and approximately the size of virus particles. Propagation in tissue culture appears to have been successful on one occasion, but difficulty has been experienced in repeating this observation. The true nature of these small particles is unknown and further study is required before deciding on their significance or possible role in regard to the origin of adenomas. In the meantime, the granules represent the only difference noted so far between the adenomatous tumors from polyposis patients and nonpolyposis patients.

5
relationship to carcinoma

a) General Factors

1) Incidence. Since it seems probable that most, if not all, carcinomas of the colon and rectum arise in preexisting benign adenomas (Morson & Bussey 1970), it is not surprising that in adenomatosis coli, with its hundreds of adenomas, there should be a high incidence of associated intestinal malignancy. Of the 617 patients in this survey, 412 (66.8%) are known to have had intestinal cancer (Table 6). If, however, the call-up group is excluded because these patients were in the main prevented by surgery from developing cancer, the cancer incidence rate of the remainder is 394 out of 500 (78.8%). It is difficult to believe that the other 20% of polyposis patients would not also have had cancer if they had lived long enough without operation. It is a fact of particular clinical significance that no less than 194 (66.2%) of the 293 presenting because of symptoms already had malignant disease.

2) Sex ratio. The 412 patients with carcinoma comprised 213 males (51.7%) and 199 females (48.3%). The Registrar General's figures for cancer of the large intestine in the general population vary from year to year but in 1936 the ratio was 5,641 males (52.7%) to 5,061 females (47.3%): in 1963 it was 6,502 males (45.1%) and 7,924 females (54.9%).

3) Age at diagnosis. The nearest estimate that can be given for the age at onset of cancer in polyposis is that of the age at diagnosis of malignant cases and, here again, it is the propositus group that supplies the most reliable information. The analysis of this group by age is given in Table 7. The average age at diagnosis was 39.9 years for males and 38.3 years for females, with 39.2 years for the whole group. In both sexes half the patients had been diagnosed by 40 years of age.

The call-up group included 11 patients who had cancer when polyposis was first diagnosed and a further 7 patients who developed malignancy after polyps had been found and who either refused surgery or had it postponed. The average age at diagnosis of cancer in these 18 persons was 37.4 years.

Table 6. Incidence rate of intestinal carcinoma in various groups of polyposis patients

Group	Total number	At diagnosis of polyposis		Later	Total	
					Number with cancer	
Indeterminate group	207	178	86.0%	2	180	87.0%
Propositus group	293	194	66.2%	20	214	73.0%
Call-up group	117	11	9.4%	7	18	15.4%
TOTAL	617	383	62.0%	29	412	66.8%

Table 7. Age distribution of patients with both polyposis coli and intestinal cancer. Propositus group (214 cases)

Age group	Males No.	%	females No.	%	Total No.	%
10	—	—	—	—	—	—
15	1	0.9	—	—	1	0.5
20	8	7.1	6	6.5	14	6.9
25	16	14.3	16	17.3	32	15.8
30	15	13.4	17	18.5	32	15.8
35	19	16.9	17	18.5	36	17.7
40	18	16.0	11	12.0	29	14.2
45	17	15.2	15	16.3	32	15.8
50	7	6.3	5	5.4	12	5.9
55	5	4.5	3	3.3	8	3.4
60	3	2.7	—	—	3	1.5
65	1	0.9	1	1.1	2	1.0
70	1	0.9	1	1.1	2	1.0
75	1	0.9	—	—	1	0.5
80	—	—	—	—	—	—
Not known	7		3		10	
TOTAL	119		95		214	
Average age	39.9 years		38.3 years		39.2 years	

The average age at which intestinal cancer was diagnosed in 5,046 nonpolyposis patients at St. Mark's Hospital was 60.3 years, with a significant difference in the ages of the two groups of about 20 years.

4) Age at death from carcinoma and polyposis. Since most patients in the propositus group had been subjected to surgery with modification of the natural course of the disease, the indeterminate group, being composed mainly of an older generation when surgery was both less frequent and less effective, was more useful in assessing

Table 8. Age distribution at death of polyposis patients with associated intestinal cancer. Indeterminate group (180 cases)

Age group	Males		Females		Total	
	No.	%	No.	%	No.	%
10	—	—	—	—	—	—
15	—	—	—	—	—	—
20	3	4.0	3	3.4	6	3.7
25	8	10.8	6	6.9	14	8.6
30	13	17.3	14	16.1	27	16.7
35	13	17.3	15	17.3	28	17.3
40	17	22.7	15	17.3	32	19.7
45	10	13.3	8	9.2	18	11.1
50	4	5.3	16	18.4	20	12.3
55	1	1.3	5	5.7	6	3.9
60	3	4.0	4	4.6	7	4.3
65	2	2.7	1	1.1	3	1.8
70	1	1.3	—	—	1	0.6
75	—	—	—	—		
80	—	—	—	—		
Not known	10		8		18	
TOTAL	85		95		180	
Average age	40.8 years		42.7 years		41.8 years	

the age distribution at death (Table 8). For males the average span of life was 40.8 years and for females 42.7 years, with an overall figure of 41.8 years. Thus, those patients succumbing to cancer did so on an average 2.6 years after the malignant tumor was diagnosed.

The average age at death is much below that for nonpolyposis patients in the general population, which for 17,016 intestinal cancer cases reported by the Registrar General in 1948 was 68.5 years and for 14,426 cases in 1963 70.4 years. There is an approximate difference of 25 years between the two figures for fatal intestinal cancer in the general population and the polyposis group. This difference is shown in the age distribution curves in Figure 40. Nearly 75% of the polyposis patients with associated malignancy had died before the age of 50, whereas less than 6% of persons with intestinal cancer in the general population were dead before that age.

b) Pathological Factors

All colectomy specimens were scrutinized for macroscopic evidence of malignancy. In the majority of instances this took the form of the usual flat, shallow ulcer with everted edges, but the polyps, particularly the larger ones, were also examined for evidence of

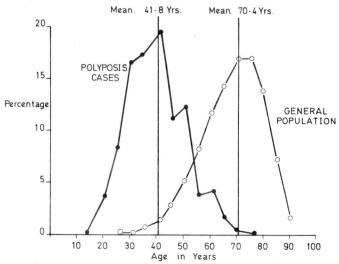

Fig. 40. Comparison of the age distribution at death from intestinal cancer of polyposis patients with that of the general population of England and Wales in the year 1963.

induration or superficial ulceration. Cancers, when found, were subjected to the routine examination applied to all malignant tumors in the Pathology Department of St. Mark's Hospital. This includes the taking of sections through the margins of the carcinoma in order to obtain possible evidence of adenomatous origin and also of venous invasion. Further sections through the area of deepest invasion determine the extent of spread by direct continuity. A dissection of the mesentery is also carried out, with removal and sectioning of all lymph nodes found. These are charted on an accurate natural-sized map, those subsequently found on microscopic examination to contain carcinoma being blacked in (Fig. 41). The growth is then graded histologically and classified by Dukes's method (Dukes 1932).

In reviewing the histology of the polyposis cases it was found that sections were available from the cancers in 148 patients and pathological reports in another 16 cases. Full information was not always obtained, but when applicable the details available have been used in the following analysis.

1. Multiplicity of Carcinomas

Major surgery was performed in 151 of the 164 patients referred to above and examination of the specimens revealed the presence of

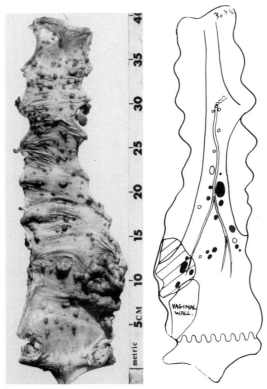

Fig. 41. Method used to report the extent of
spread of cancer when associated with
polyposis coli. *Left:* Surface view of
specimen removed by synchronous
combined excision. A carcinoma and 260
polyps are present. *Right:* Drawing of the
mesenteric aspect of the specimen, showing
the carcinoma in relation to the peritoneal
reflexion and the dentate line. Twenty-four
lymph nodes were removed for microscopic
examination and 16 were found to contain
metastases (marked in black).

more than one carcinoma in 67, the highest number in any specimen
being 7. Eleven patients whose specimens originally showed only
one cancer subsequently developed a further cancer in the residual
large intestine, making a total of 78 individuals with multiple
cancers, or 47.6%.

In a survey of 6,309 patients with intestinal cancer, unassociated
with polyposis, treated at St. Mark's Hospital in the period 1928–65,
164 (2.6%) had more than one cancer simultaneously, and another

82 (1.3%) developed metachronous carcinoma, the total incidence of multiple intestinal cancers being 3.9% (Bussey et al. 1967). Multiple cancers were thus twelve times more frequently encountered in polyposis patients than among members of the general population suffering from intestinal cancer.

2. Extent of Spread—Dukes's Classification

Dukes (1932) subdivided intestinal cancers into three groups.

A cases   Those where the growth has spread by direct continuity into the submucosa and/or muscle coat, but not beyond, and where there is no lymphatic involvement.

B cases   In this group there is spread beyond the muscle coat into the perirectal tissues, but still without lymphatic involvement.

C cases   In these tumors metastasis to the lymph nodes has occurred.

Bussey, Dukes, and Lockhart-Mummery (1960) gave the proportions of these three groups in a series of 2,037 excision specimens as: A cases, 15.2%; B cases, 33.9%; C cases, 50.9%. In 69 polyposis operation specimens with one cancer there were 25 A, 19 B, and 25 C cases. A further 55 specimens contained more than one carcinoma, and if the group of the most advanced growth present is taken, these comprise 4 A, 16 B, and 35 C cases. The total for the whole 124 cases is, therefore:

A cases	29	23.4
B cases	35	28.2
C cases	60	48.4

The differences in proportion of A, B, and C cases between the general series of intestinal cancer and the polyposis group with malignancy are not significant.

3. Grade of Malignancy

It is the practice at St. Mark's Hospital to subdivide intestinal cancer into three grades on the basis of histology.

(i) *Low grade of malignancy (well-differentiated).*

In these tumors there is a well-preserved glandular pattern closely resembling that of normal mucosa, the cells lining the tubules usually being arranged in orderly layers 2 to 3 cells in thickness. The cells and their nuclei are generally of uniform size and mitoses are uncommon.

Table 9. Proportions of cancers of low, average, and high grades of malignancy in polyposis patients and the general population

| Grade | Intestinal Cancer in | | | |
| | Polyposis cases | | General population | |
	No.	%	No.	%
Low	57	25.0	407	19.4
Average	147	64.5	1,266	60.4
High	24	10.5	424	20.2
TOTAL	228		2,097	

(ii) *Average grade of malignancy (moderately differentiated).*

Tubule formation is still prominent in this group. The tubules are seldom of the normal round or oval type, but are irregular and tortuous in nature and lined by multiple layers of cells. Mitoses are common and cells and nuclei show an increasing degree of irregularity in size and shape.

(iii) *High grade of malignancy (poorly differentiated).*

The glandular pattern of these growths is either of a very primitive character or entirely absent, the tumor consisting chiefly of isolated cells or small clumps arranged chaotically. Pleomorphism of the cells is a noticeable feature and irregular mitoses commonly occur.

A total of 286 malignant tumors of the large intestine was distributed among the 164 polyposis patients with cancer. In 58 tumors there was no evidence on which to make a histological grading, but the grading of the other 228 tumors is set out in Table 9, together with that of a larger series of intestinal cancers in the general population. The main difference is that there are fewer high grade carcinomas in polyposis patients. Among those under the age of 30 years the proportion of high grade cancers is only about 12%, as compared with a corresponding figure of 53.4% in nonpolyposis cases (Recio & Bussey 1965).

4. Distribution of Intestinal Cancer

Comparison of the regional distribution of carcinoma in the large intestine in polyposis cases and in a series from the general population reported by Smiddy and Goligher (1957) is made in Table 10. The distributions are generally similar in the two series, and there is no significance in the minor differences.

The occurrence within a short interval of several cecal carcinomas

Table 10. Comparison of site distribution of cancer of the large intestine in polyposis and nonpolyposis patients

Site	Polyposis series		General population series (Smiddy & Goligher 1957)	
	No.	%	No.	%
Cecum	13	4.9	101	6.1
Ascending colon	4	1.5	48	2.9
Hepatic flexure	8	3.0	29	1.8
Transverse colon	18	6.9	77	4.7
Splenic flexure	16	6.1	50	3.0
Left colon	63	24.0	395	24.0
Rectum	141	53.6	944	57.5
Unclassified	23			
TOTAL	286		1,644	

Table 11. Relationship of age and site of carcinoma in polyposis patients

Site	No. of cases	Average age (years)
Cecum	13	52.2
Ascending colon	4	43.8
Hepatic flexure	8	44.9
Transverse colon	18	42.9
Splenic flexure	16	42.2
Left colon	63	37.3
Rectum	141	39.0
TOTAL	263	

in polyposis patients of rather more than usually mature age suggested an investigation into the age of onset of cancer at different sites with the results shown in Table 11. The trend is for cancer of the right half of the colon to arise at a later age than in the left colon or rectum.

5. Origin of Carcinoma in Adenomatous Tumors

As with solitary adenomas, the adenomas of polyposis coli can be arranged in a sequence, beginning with those showing slight epithelial dysplasia, through successive phases of increasing histological irregularity, to those which have undergone frank malignant degeneration. Classification of the two extremes presents no difficulty, but the intermediate stages are variously interpreted as "carcinoma in situ," "preinvasive carcinoma," or "carcinoma at an early stage." The polyp illustrated in Figure 42 is a typical example of this lesion.

Most of the tumor is adenomatous, in sharp contrast with the appearances in the central region, which are those of carcinoma in every respect except that of definite invasion. There is increased stratification of the epithelium, bridging of the acini, irregularity in the shape and size of the cells, and greater mitotic activity (Fig. 43). For such tumors "carcinoma in situ" or "preinvasive carcinoma" are perhaps useful terms, provided that they are intended to denote a tumor at the final stage of becoming malignant, rather than the first stage of a definite carcinoma, since they may still be regarded as clinically benign. Invasion across the line of the muscularis mucosa introduces a new and more dangerous threat to the patient's well-being, namely, the possibility of lymphatic spread. In the absence of exact histological criteria to differentiate "benign" from "malignant" tumors, invasion of the muscularis mucosa at least provides a distinctive step at which malignancy may be said to have occurred (Morson & Bussey 1970; Morson 1973). At St. Mark's Hospital tumors in which there is no such invasion are not classified among cases of malignancy. Macroscopical and microscopically appearances of definite invasive carcinoma arising in a preexisting adenoma are shown in Figures 44 and 45.

The fact that benign adenomatous tissue is found at the margin of an intestinal cancer is strong circumstantial evidence that the cancer arose in a preexisting benign tumor. When a similar combination of benign and malignant tissue is found in a polyposis specimen, it could be argued that the cancer is invading an adjacent adenoma, and it is not possible in every instance to refute this. For this reason some caution is needed when making a comparison of the incidence of benign origin of cancer in polyposis with that of nonpolyposis cases.

No histology was available in 87 (30.4%) of the 286 cancers present, but of the remaining 199, 72 showed the presence of adenomatous growth at the margin of the carcinoma, i.e., 36.2%. For specimens examined at St. Mark's Hospital the proportion was slightly greater (49 in 131 carcinomas, or 37.4%).

With cancers from nonpolyposis patients it has been found that 10.6% show evidence of adenomatous tissue at the margin, suggesting an origin in a preexisting benign tumor (Morson 1966). It was also shown that the proportion of such cases varied inversely with the extent of local spread. The increase in the polyposis cases is thus probably due partly to earlier diagnosis and partly to the larger number of cases of multiple cancers, some of which were at an earlier stage of development before the original adenoma had been destroyed by the carcinoma.

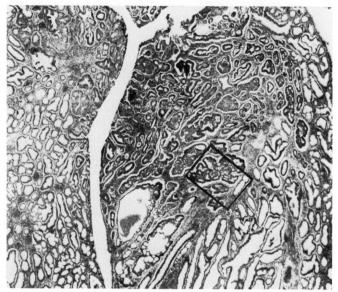

Fig. 42. Part of an adenomatous polyp containing an area of
irregular glandular pattern which could be described as
"severe dysplasia." The marked area is shown at greater
magnification in Fig. 43. (×25) (Reduced by 30%)

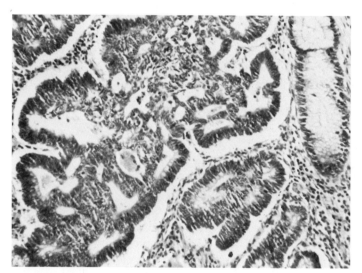

Fig. 43. High power view of the area marked in Fig. 42.
Hyperchromatism, acinar bridging, nuclear irregularity, and
other features of malignancy are present, but there is no
definite evidence of invasion. (×200) (Reduced by 40%)

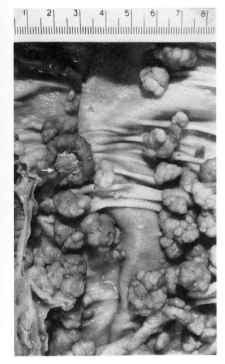

Fig. 44. Adenomatous tumor with ulcerated center where malignant change has taken place.

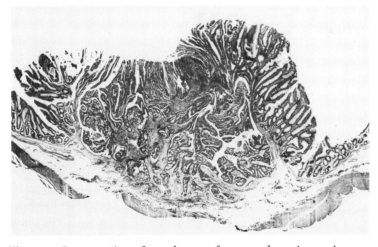

Fig. 45. Cross-section of an adenoma from a polyposis specimen. The central region is occupied by adenocarcinoma that is invading the submucosa. (×18) (Reduced by 30%)

6. Survival Rate

One or more carcinomas were present in 54 of the 138 major operation specimens removed at St. Mark's Hospital. Three of these patients died at operation, and analysis shows that the 51 operation survivors had a crude five-year survival rate of 58.3%, or, when adjusted for age and death from other causes, a corrected survival rate of 60.4%. The corresponding rates for cancer of the rectum in the general population are 48.3% and 57.5% respectively.

The comparisons that have been made above between cancer in polyposis and nonpolyposis patients show few differences. These include an increase in the number of cases of multiple cancer, an earlier onset of cancer, and an earlier age of death in polyposis cancer patients. In all other respects malignant disease of the large intestine supervening on familial polyposis coli is indistinguishable from that derived from other sources.

6
associated lesions

1. GARDNER'S SYNDROME

In 1951 Gardner reported a family in which seven members suffered from a combination of lesions consisting of:
a. adenomatosis of the large intestine;
b. multiple osteomata of the skull and mandible;
c. multiple epidermoid cysts and soft tissue tumors of the skin.
This syndrome, which now bears his name, was elaborated upon by Gardner and his co-workers (Gardner & Plenk 1952; Gardner & Richards 1953) and by a follow-up study of the family (Gardner 1962). Similar cases had been reported previously (Devic & Bussy 1912; Cabot 1935; Fitzgerald 1943) and so many subsequently that Gardner's syndrome now has a very large bibliography of an increasingly confused and controversial nature. It is certain that many of the cases reported under his name would be rejected by Gardner owing to the absence of some of the features described as well as to the inclusion of extraneous lesions. Gardner enlarged the syndrome when he reviewed the family several years later (Gardner 1962; 1969). By then abnormal dentition had been noted. This included impacted supernumerary and permanent teeth, unusually early caries and loss of teeth (most affected members of the family over 20 years of age had dentures), dentigerous cysts, and abnormal bone structure of the mandible. Desmoid tumors, both of the abdominal wall operation scars and intra-abdominally in the mesentery of the small intestine had also been observed. These are described in more detail below. The more obvious osteomas of the skull and mandible had been reinforced by similar tumors in the long bones and elsewhere.

The surface lesions of Gardner's syndrome are sometimes useful pointers to the possible presence of polyposis. In particular, the epidermoid cysts and osteomas may exist for many years before the intestinal polyps give rise to symptoms. Certainly their occurrence in a member of a polyposis coli family is an indication for sigmoidoscopic examination. Moreover, epidermoid cysts may lead to the discovery of unexpected polyposis. The term "sebaceous cyst" has been used for a group of cysts of differing types and origins, which include the pilar cyst (the common wen), the epidermoid cyst, and those found in steatocystoma multiplex. Leppard (1974) has investigated the "sebaceous cysts" associated with Gardner's syndrome and finds that all those examined histologically are epidermoid cysts. Thus wens and steatocystoma multiplex are not indicative of associated polyposis. Moreover, she suggests that although epidermoid cysts are common in the general population, they are very uncommon before the age of puberty, and their observation under this age should be followed by sigmoidoscopy to ascertain whether intestinal polyps are also present.

Other lesions that have been put forward for recognition but that have not as yet received official blessing include carcinoma of the thyroid (Crail 1949; Camiel et al. 1968), carcinoma of the ampulla of Vater and duodenum (Cabot 1935; MacDonald et al. 1967; Capps et al. 1968; McFarland et al. 1968), adrenal cancer (Marshall et al. 1967), adenomas of the small intestine (Kaplan 1961; Chiat et al. 1962; Heald 1967), carcinoid tumors of the small intestine (Hayes et al. 1959; Heald 1967), tumors of the brain and central nervous system (see under "Turcot's syndrome"), skin pigmentation (Weston & Weiner 1967), and lymphoid polyps of the ileum (Thomford & Greenberger 1968). Of this list the periampullary carcinomas may perhaps have prior claim to recognition.

a) Periampullary Carcinoma

At least 20 cases of carcinoma of the duodenum, ampulla of Vater, or pancreas are known to exist. These include 14 males and 6 females. The age range is 18 to 60 years, with an average of 40.9 years. The interval of time between colectomy and diagnosis of the ampullary carcinoma varied from 1 to 25 years; average about 12 years. Four of the cases have occurred in patients operated on at St. Mark's Hospital, representing about 4% of all patients surviving colectomy for 5 years and 12% of patients with possible Gardner's syndrome (Bussey 1972). Another patient died 10 months after colectomy for nonmalignant polyposis. Death was due to generalized carcinomatosis of the abdominal cavity. The primary site could not be determined, and although this was suspected to be in the periampullary region, confirmation was impossible, as permission for postmorten examination could not be obtained. Most of these 20 patients had at least some of the other signs of Gardner's syndrome.

b) Desmoid tumors

The osteomas, epidermal cysts, and subcutaneous fibromas of Gardner's syndrome have little clinical significance other than their possible value as pointers to polyposis. Desmoid tumors, on the other hand, may be of concern to the clinician and a danger to the patient. The tumors usually arise between 1 and 3 years after surgery for polyposis, either in the abdominal wall or intra-abdominally, mostly in the mesentery of the small intestine (Shepherd 1958; Gorlin & Chaudry 1960; McAdam & Goligher 1970). They may become very large, like one removed at the Mayo Clinic that measured 30 cms by 36 cms by 15 cms and weighed over 3,800 grams (Simpson et al. 1964). Not infrequently the tumors are multiple, and removal may be followed by further desmoid formation. Occasionally they precede the discovery of polyposis. One patient, who underwent cholecystectomy at 19 years of age, developed a desmoid in the abdominal scar three years later. It was not until he was 54 years of age that polyposis was diagnosed. In most patients the desmoids are preceded by surgical trauma, but this was not the case in two patients. In one of these the trauma of childbirth might have been the cause: the other case was a girl of 16, admitted for what was thought to be an ovarian cyst, which on laparotomy proved to be an enormous desmoid tumor involving the transverse colon. Polyposis was diagnosed two years later.

Smith (1959) found desmoid tumors in 7 (3.5%) of 201 polyposis patients at the Mayo Clinic and stated "this is certainly several hundredfold the incidence complicating operations in unselected series." The proportion is a little higher in the St. Mark's Hospital series, where 8 out of 141 patients (5.7%) operated on subsequently developed desmoids. In the whole series of 617 patients, 26 desmoids were reported (4.2%), but this is certainly an underestimate.

Histologically desmoid tumors are generally regarded as benign fibromata, though at the margin the fibroblasts infiltrate locally into the neighboring tissues, sometimes diagnosed as a fibrosarcoma of low-grade malignancy. Clinically they are commonly thought to be carcinomatous recurrences in those patients who had associated malignant disease. Laparotomy reveals their true nature, but even so the intra-abdominal desmoids are frequently inoperable owing to extensive involvement of the root of the mesentery. Left in situ, they do not grow indefinitely but appear to reach an optimum size and then remain static. The main threat to the patient's well-being is that of mechanical obstruction of the intestine or the urinary tract. Two patients in the Register with irremovable mesenteric fibromata have each remained well for almost fifteen years. Altogether 12 patients with mesenteric desmoids are recorded in the St. Mark's Hospital Register, and at least 35 have been reported elsewhere. Death in 7 patients appears to have been due basically to the abdominal fibroma, but in most of these patients there had been previous surgery to remove the tumor.

In a few reports, no definite tumor was present, but a condition that is described as "diffuse fibrous infiltration" of the mesentery (Simpson et al. 1964). It has also been observed that intestinal obstruction due to dense fibrous bands appears to be more common following polyposis operations than after surgery for other intestinal diseases (Lockhart-Mummery 1967). The complications of postoperative fibromas, generalized fibromatosis, and fibrous adhesions all seem to be one aspect of the general tissue growth postulated by Smith (1968).

The incidence and nature of Gardner's syndrome. It is unlikely that anyone else has observed a family like Gardner's Kindred 109, and he may well have been fortunate in this respect. Certainly no similar family appears in the St. Mark's Hospital series. In some families several members may each have some but not all of the expected features. In general, it is easier to state that a family shows the syndrome rather than that individual members have it.

In 50 of the families in the St. Mark's Register there was at least one member with at least one lesion of Gardner's syndrome in addition to the polyps, but this might be considered too low a standard on which to diagnose the syndrome. There were, however, twenty families containing between two and nine individuals with some of the features of the syndrome, and if these are accepted as genuine examples, the incidence rate among polyposis families in which more than one member has polyposis is 18.2%. The incidence of solitary patients with possible Gardner's syndrome among this group of families is 14.6% and among polyposis patients without a family history the proportion with possible Gardner's syndrome is 15.6%. It must be kept in mind that investigations to confirm the presence or absence of all the stigmata of Gardner's syndrome are not always carried out, and many examples undoubtedly go unrecorded.

Another controversial issue is the genetic aspect of the syndrome. The question whether or not all its features result from a single dominant gene, as Gardner believes, or are two or more genes involved, has not been satisfactorily resolved. McKusick (1962) has stated that the type of polyposis in Gardner's syndrome differs from the non-Gardner's type in that the polyps are more scattered and the mucosa less carpeted. There is little support for this in the St. Mark's

Hospital cases, where there is a wide variation in the number of polyps present in the colons removed from patients both with and without the other indications of the syndrome. Nor is it generally true that the polyps of Gardner's syndrome, like those of the Peutz–Jeghers syndrome, can occur anywhere in the gastrointestinal tract (Colcock & Zomorodian 1966). A few cases of gastric and small intestinal polyps are reported, though little is known of the histology of these extracolonic tumors. One St. Mark's Hospital patient had polyposis coli, epidermoid cysts, subcutaneous fibromas, carcinoma of the ampulla of Vater and gastric polypi, but these were not adenomas but hamartomas. Smith (1959) gives his view of the various reports of Gardner's syndrome when he says: "It seems most likely that the syndrome described by Gardner is the full-blown manifestation of a spectrum of pathological changes which could affect, in variable numbers and combination, *any* patient with multiple polyposis." He believes also that "a single mutation is responsible for most of the various syndromes associated with multiple colonic polyposis."

The idea that all adenomatous polyposis may be Gardner's syndrome with different degrees of manifestation of the subsidiary lesions is interesting. Certainly, the more these are looked for the more they are found. Utsunomiya and Nakamura (1974) find a high incidence of nodules of increased bone opacity in the mandibles of polyposis patients and an absence of such lesions in patients with a few adenomas only or those with the Peutz–Jeghers syndrome. If these nodules are a further extension of the osteomatous disease noted by Gardner, this observation would be evidence of a much wider distribution of the syndrome among polyposis patients. Obviously, the polyposis families require investigation in greater depth for longer periods before definite solutions can be given to the many problems involved.

c) Turcot's Syndrome

Association of polyposis coli with malignant tumors of the central nervous system in two members of a family has been reported (Turcot et al. 1959). A boy of 15 years was found to have polyposis and carcinoma of the colon. He died two years later with medulloblastoma of the spinal cord. His sister, aged 13, was also diagnosed as suffering from polyposis, colectomy being carried out at 16 years of age. About five years later a cerebral tumor was discovered, but death occurred suddenly before treatment could be started, and a glioblastoma of the frontal lobe was found at postmortem examination. This seems to be the only familial instance recorded, though two other individuals are reported (Crail 1949; Camiel et al. 1968) and there is one case in the present series. This was the son of a polyposis patient who at 14 years was found on routine examination to have a few sessile polyps and after two and a half years died from a medulloblastoma of the cerebellum. In another St. Mark's family a son died at 24 years from a cerebral medulloblastoma, but there was no evidence that he had ever been examined for polyposis, although this might have developed later had he lived. In view of the few recorded examples of Turcot's syndrome and the early age of onset of both polyposis and brain tumors, it is possible that this association has little significance. On the other hand, it may be a further example of the unusual tumor associations found in Gardner's syndrome.

d) Associated Polypoid Conditions

The various diseases that affect the gastrointestinal tract, and by manifesting themselves as multiple polypoid lesions have simulated adenomatosis, are dealt with in Chapter 9, "Differential diagnosis." Two such conditions, however, deserve notice here as associated lesions because of possible genetic linkages, though a general description is deferred. These are multiple juvenile polyposis and "minor" or "recessive" adenomatous polyposis.

1) **"Minor" or "Recessive" adenomatous polyposis.** Veale studied the polyposis families in the St. Mark's Hospital Polyposis Register and also any familial pattern of adenomatous and carcinomatous tumors of the large intestine. He concluded that it was probable that all adenomas, whether present singly, or as a few, or several, or in the hundreds, as in polyposis, have a genetic origin. On this basis he conceived a genetic model to explain the varied incidence and behavior in these different conditions (Veale 1965). This is dealt with in the section on "Differential Diagnosis," but mention is made here of the importance, if this theory is correct, of distinguishing between the dominant and recessive forms of inheritance. The suggestion is made that the number of adenomas present can be used as a standard, 100 being a possible dividing line.

2) **Multiple juvenile polyposis.** In 1966, Veale and his co-workers reported a series of patients with juvenile polyposis, among whom was a girl of 13 years whose father was said to have had adenomatous polyposis. Since then a review of the tumors removed from the father showed these to consist mainly of juvenile polyps, with only a few adenomas. Some years later he underwent an excision for

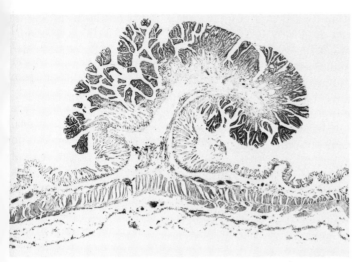

Fig. 46. Adenoma of terminal ileum. This is the only example of benign epithelial tumor of the small intestine found in association with adenomatous polyposis at St. Mark's Hospital. (×10) (Reduced by 35%)

"polyposis coli and carcinoma of the rectum," though this diagnosis is now in dispute. Two other families are known where juvenile and adenomatous polyps are believed to exist in different siblings, but which cannot be confirmed owing to the inability to obtain histological proof of the adenomatous polyps. It is still possible that the two types of polyposis may exist in different members of the same family. There is almost certainly some kind of genetic linkage with adenomas, the exact nature of which will only be found on observation of more cases.

e) Other Associated Lesions

Most of the lesions reported at various times as being associated with polyposis have been mentioned under "Gardner's syndrome." One point may be elaborated here. For practical purposes it may be dogmatically stated that the adenomas of polyposis do not extend into the small intestine. It has already been mentioned that apparent extension into the ileum proves on investigation to be lymphoid hyperplasia. However, it must be admitted that in about 170 colectomy specimens examined there has been one example of true adenoma of the ileum (Fig. 46). A small carcinoid tumor of the ileum was also present (Heald 1967). A second case of adenoma of the small intestine is known among the patients recorded in the Register, and there is also a patient who had a small villous adenoma arising from her ileostomy. Chiat et al. (1962) and Kaplan (1961) also reported one case each of what appears to be a genuine adenoma of the duodenum. Such instances are extremely rare and in each case the small bowel tumor appears to be solitary. Hoffmann and Goligher (1971) have reported three polyposis patients in whom polyps of the stomach and duodenum were also present and called attention to fifteen other reported cases. One patient, operated on at St. Mark's Hospital for carcinoma of the ampulla of Vater, was found to have polyps of the stomach and duodenum, but histologically these tumors were hamartomas (Parks, Bussey, & Lockhart-Mummery 1970). The significance of these findings is not known.

7
the natural course of
adenomatous polyposis coli

Four stages can be recognized in the inception and progress of adenomatosis coli:

1. development of the adenomas;
2. appearance of symptoms;
3. malignant degeneration in one or more adenomas;
4. death from malignant disease.

1. DEVELOPMENT OF THE ADENOMAS

a) Time of Appearance

Although the disease is frequently referred to as "congenital polyposis," there is no evidence that adenomas have ever been present at birth. There are few reports of the tumors being found in patients under the age of 10 years, and it has to be remembered that multiple juvenile polyposis has a much earlier onset than the adenomatosis for which it has been mistaken. Conversely, there are many examples of sigmoidoscopic examination that gave a positive diagnosis only after a series of negative results.

The age distribution at the time of diagnosis of adenomatosis in the propositus group of the St. Mark's Hospital series has been shown in Figure 2. The range was from 4 to 72 years and the mean age was 35.8 years. By contrast the mean age at diagnosis in the 117 patients in the call-up group was 24.5 years and the range from 9 to 57 years. It would appear from this comparison that, in general, polyps exist for at least ten years before giving rise to symptoms sufficiently severe to cause the patient to seek medical advice. However, some patients as yet unaffected will develop adenomas in the second half of life, and when these are eventually recorded the difference between the propositus and call-up groups will be somewhat less.

In an endeavor to pinpoint more definitely the actual time at which polyps appear, a search was made for patients who had been without polyps when first examined sigmoidoscopically, but who developed these later. Twenty-one such patients were found. The estimated ages at which adenomas appeared ranged from 11 to 47.5 years, the average age being 22.2 years, about 2 years less than that of the main call-up group.

These figures are based on the 617 patients surveyed in the present series. The youngest age at which polyps were diagnosed was about 4 years and the next earliest 9 years and 3 months. Polyposis in the first decade of life has been reported elsewhere. Abramson (1967) diagnosed polyps that were undoubtedly adenomas in a boy of 6 years. McKenney (1936) in his family found polyps in four siblings at ages 2, 5, 9, and 11 years. A section of a rectal biopsy taken from a baby of 9 months, a child of a polyposis patient, has also been seen. Though no polyps were visible in the rectum there was an area of adenomatous proliferation in the biopsy. These examples of early development of adenomas must be regarded as exceptional. At the other end of the scale, the latest known onset of polyps in the St. Mark's Hospital series was somewhere between 42 and 53 years of age, though more extreme examples can be found in the literature, such as that reported by Knapp (1965). The mother of eleven children, six of whom suffered from polyposis, was herself examined both by proctoscopy and double contrast enema at the age of 70 years with negative results. Four years later she developed cancer of the rectum and at operation was found to have had polyposis as well.

b) Mode of Appearance of Polyps

A study of the clinical histories of adenomatous patients suggests that in the majority of cases the onset of the tumors is a slow and insidious process. The first sign of the disease seen on sigmoidoscopic examination is usually recorded in some such phrase as "two or three small polyps in rectum" or "? mucosal nodules." In some cases little or no change may be observed at first, with only a slow growth of polyps over a number of years. One patient, for instance, was called-up at 30 years of age; he was symptomless and a few polyps only were seen. Twelve years later the polypi were said "to be increasing, but still not many," and a further two years passed with little change. However, the x-ray appearances suggested (incorrectly) possible malignant change and colectomy was performed. On the other hand the early report of a few polyps only may in some cases be followed within a year or two by the observation of "large numbers of polyps seen."

2. SYMPTOMS

Accurate information about symptoms and time of onset is not easily obtained. Full or partial case histories were available for 293 patients, 196 of which were from the propositus group and 97 from the call-up group. The average age of onset of symptoms in the propositus patients was 32.9 years and, since the mean age at diagnosis was 35.8 years, symptoms were on the average present for about three years. Of the 97 call-up patients studied, only 27 had any symptoms, the average age being 25.5 years. The 70 call-up patients who claimed to have no symptoms had an average age of 24.8 years when their polyposis was diagnosed.

The main symptoms were:

1. **Bleeding.** More than three-quarters of the presenting patients (78.9%) complained of rectal bleeding that had lasted on average for about two-and-a-half years. Curiously, although nearly two-thirds of this group had associated cancer, this had little effect on the results, the proportion with bleeding being a little less, but the bleeding having been present for a slightly longer time. Among those with symptoms, the percentage of call-up cases with bleeding was rather more than for the propositus group (87%).
2. **Diarrhea.** About 70% of the patients in the propositus group suffered with diarrhea, again for an average period of about two and a half years, but for the noncancer patients the proportion was 63.0% as against 79.6% for polyposis cancer patients. Diarrhea was also present in three-quarters of the call-up group with symptoms, but had been present less than two years.
3. **Pain.** Pain, mostly abdominal in character and only rarely rectal, anal, or sacral, was present in about 40% of the propositus group.
4. **Other symptoms.** Mucous discharge was mentioned in about 30% of cases and constipation in only 4%. The disease was discovered in 13 patients as the result of an acute emergency, 8 with intestinal obstruction, 2 with peritonitis following perforation of a colonic carcinoma, 1 with severe hemorrhage, and 2 dying with carcinomatosis. A further patient might be included under this heading, as his polyposis was discovered at postmortem examination following a road accident.

Intussusception did not appear in any of the available clinical histories, nor did obstruction in any of the younger patients without cancer, though these symptoms are commonly encountered in Peutz–Jeghers polyposis.

3. ONSET OF CANCER

The average age at diagnosis of cancer in polyposis has been given in Chapter 5, "Relationship to carcinoma" as 39.2 years, which is about three years after diagnosis of polyps, six years after the onset of symptoms, and some 14 to 15 years after the appearance of polyps. The age range was 18 to 79 years. In approximately 7,000 cases of intestinal cancer in nonpolyposis patients at St. Mark's Hospital, the range was 17 to 94 years, though it is known that younger cases have been reported. The youngest intestinal cancer patient known personally was a boy aged 10 years. Similarly, though the youngest polyposis case with cancer in the St. Mark's series was aged 18 years, younger examples have been recorded. McKenney (1939) observed in the family he studied the fatal outcome of carcinoma in a boy of 15 years. Coleman and Eckert (1956) described five carcinomas in a colectomy specimen from a boy of 13 and Capps et al. (1968) reported a similar number of malignant growths in a patient aged 14. As with the early appearance of adenomas, such cases are exceptional, but since they are known to exist it is the practice at St. Mark's Hospital, when informing patients that their children need not be examined before the age of 14 years, to add that should any intestinal symptoms appear before that time the children should be brought up for examination immediately.

4. AGE AT DEATH FROM CANCER

As has been shown in "Relationship to carcinoma" (Chapter 5), the nearest estimate that can be given for the age at death from cancer following polyposis, in the absence of medical treatment, is that based on the indeterminate group and is an average of 42.0 years.

One may sum up the natural course of familial polyposis coli in the average untreated patient by tabulating the passage of the main milestones in the disease as follows:

Age of appearance of adenomas	24.5 years
Age of onset of symptoms	33.0 years
Age of diagnosis of adenomas	35.8 years
Age of diagnosis of cancer	39.2 years
Age at death from cancer	42.0 years

8
treatment

Surgery is the only effective treatment at the present moment and is basically directed at the removal of the adenomas in order to prevent cancerous degeneration. Theoretically, this aim is best achieved by excision of the whole large intestine (total proctocolectomy), but this leaves the patient with the permanent handicap of an ileostomy. Many surgeons, however, favor the retention of a normal bowel function by resection of the whole colon accompanied by ileorectal anastomosis (ileoproctostomy) and diathermy destruction of the rectal polyps. This latter course imposes an obligation on both patient and surgeon in respect of the retained rectum. The patient must be willing to have periodic examinations of the rectum, and the surgeon must be prepared to do this and to destroy any new adenomas that have arisen. Each method has its advocates, but it will be seen that total colectomy and ileorectal anastomosis is the one preferred at St. Mark's Hospital. Obviously, if cancer has already supervened in the lower rectum, no option is available and total proctocolectomy is the only course open.

Results of Treatment at St. Mark's Hospital

From 1948 to 1973, 126 patients underwent surgery for polyposis at St. Mark's Hospital. Miscellaneous types of operation were used in 13 patients, mainly because previous surgery had been carried out or because of the presence of hepatic metastases. Total proctocolectomy and ileostomy was performed on 22 patients, of whom 19 had cancer of the rectum. The 3 patients without malignant disease had all been operated on before the end of 1958. Half of the patients undergoing total proctocolectomy are dead, 1 with late complications after operation, one from pancreatitis three years later, and 9 from recurrent carcinoma. Nine patients are alive for periods from 12 years to nearly 22 years, the other 2 having been operated on only about 1 year and 2 years ago, respectively.

Total colectomy and ileorectal anastomosis was the operation employed in 91 cases. There were two immediate postoperative deaths and subsequently 14 other patients died from various causes; only 2 succumbed to recurrent carcinoma, although 14 of the 91 patients had also had malignant disease. The remaining 75 patients have survived for periods of a few months up to 25 years, the average being 11.3 years.

Complications of Surgery

a) Regression and recurrence of adenomas in the retained rectum. The regression of polyps in the rectum following colectomy and ileorectal anastomosis has been observed in some patients. This was first reported by Hubbard (1957), who performed this operation on a boy aged 9 years. The intention was to fulgurate the rectal polyps at a later date, but on the first sigmoidoscopy, five months after operation, there was a considerable decrease in the number of polyps observed. A second examination four months later showed only six polyps, and even these had disappeared at the end of a further two months. No fulguration of the polyps was carried out at any time, and no further polyps appeared during the next eighteen months. Similar cases have been recorded by Cole and Holden (1959), Cole et al. (1961), and Wenckert (1965). The regression does not occur in every case of ileorectal anastomosis, but appears to a marked degree in certain patients who are usually in the younger age groups.

Regression of the polyps seems to be an established fact and, if so, it is of great interest that considerable numbers of neoplastic tumors, even though benign, can reverse their normal character and disappear. This would indicate a field for the investigation of possible environmental factors and their interaction with those of genetic origin. If regression of polyps is a fact, it is almost equally certain that the phenomenon is not permanent. In most cases adenomas eventually reappear in the rectum, requiring control by diathermy, although this may not be for some years. An analysis of 62 patients followed up after colectomy shows that 34 remained free from polyps for an average period of about six years, and in a further 13 patients there were only a few polyps over the same period. Most patients in these two groups subsequently developed adenomas in increasing numbers. The remaining 15 patients had adenomas present in the rectum during most of the postcolectomy follow-up period. In the majority of patients the rate of development of the polyps appeared to decrease in the first years after colectomy.

An attempt was made to correlate the growth rate of polyps with increasing time after ileorectal anastomosis by comparing the number of diathermy treatments. Thirty-six patients have had regular supervision of the rectum for periods up to twenty years after operation. During the first ten-year period the average number of diathermy treatments per patient observed was 3.3; in the second ten years 4.6, indicating a general trend for new adenomas to appear more rapidly as time goes on. It is not known if this is due to the loss of some inhibiting factor. The possible reasons for regression have been suggested by Cole and Holden (1959) as: (1) diversion of ileal contents directly into the rectum; (2) extirpation of a major portion of the diseased organ; (3) diminution of blood supply to the rectal segment. Which, if any, of these is correct is still without confirmation.

b) **Cancer in the retained rectum.** In this series of 89 patients surviving total colectomy with ileorectal anastomosis there were 2 who subsequently developed a carcinoma of the rectum, at intervals of two years four months and six years eight months, respectively, after the first operation. Excision of the rectum was carried out, and in each case the cancer was found to be at an early stage (Dukes's A case). A third patient underwent excision of the rectum about nine and one-half years after colectomy. In spite of repeated diathermy treatment, the rectum became carpeted with confluent adenomas, and it was decided advisable to excise the stump. It is interesting that it was this patient whose original colectomy specimen showed the largest number of adenomas recorded, more than 5,000 in all.

There is a wide variation reported in the incidence of malignancy in the retained rectum. Everson and Allen (1954) reviewed 115 cases and found that 5.2% subsequently had rectal cancer. In another report (Flotte et al. 1956), the proportion was 19% (4 with subsequent carcinoma out of 21 operation survivors), which is about the same as that given by Bacon et al. (1957) in their series of 23 patients, of whom 4 developed rectal carcinoma (17.4%). The most gloomy report came from Moertel and his co-workers (1970), who found an overall figure of 22% for the proportion of patients developing rectal cancer, a figure which rises to 59% when follow-up reaches twenty-three years. For this reason they advocate total proctocolectomy for the effective control of polyposis. This conclusion is not, however, upheld by the figure published by Schaupp and Volpe (1972), who had only one case of rectal cancer in 48 patients undergoing colectomy and ileorectal anastomosis. It is certainly not supported by the present series from St. Mark's Hospital. The periods of time survived by patients who have had colectomy and ileorectal anastomosis and the number subsequently developing rectal cancer

Table 12.

Five-year period	No. of patients surviving period	No. of patients developing cancer	Risk of cancer	Cumulative risk (%)
1	64	1	$\frac{1}{65} = 1.5\%$	1.5
2	47	1	$\frac{1}{48} = 2.1\%$	3.6
3	27	nil	—	3.6
4	13	nil	—	3.6
5	2	nil	—	3.6

are shown in Table 12, where the cumulative risk is given as 3.6%. Even if the patient whose rectum was excised for uncontrollable polyposis is included, the risk is only 5.7%. This figure, taking into account the early stage at which cancer, if it supervenes, should be diagnosed, still provides justification for the more conservative operation.

Control of Cancer in Polyposis Families

The investigation and follow-up of polyposis families and the treatment of affected members has been described. The important objective is to get individuals with polyposis treated before they develop cancer. Cancer prevention has limited scope in the propositus group as two-thirds of these patients already have cancer when first seen. The incidence of malignancy among the siblings is, however, less than that found in propositus family members and even more so among the children of affected members. The records of the St. Mark's Hospital Polyposis Register show a dramatic decrease in malignant disease among call-up family members as compared with the propositus group. The latter group contains 293 patients, of whom 194 (66.2%) had carcinoma of the colon or rectum when first seen, whereas, there were only 11 patients with cancer among 117 (9.4%) found to have polyposis when called up for examination.

The degree of success achieved by the surgical treatment of patients caught before carcinoma has occurred has been demonstrated, the risk of subsequent rectal cancer being estimated at the moment as 3.6%. The resulting cancers have been discovered at a curable stage. It is justifiable to claim that where there is active follow-up of the family and willing cooperation from its members a remarkable degree of cancer control is possible.

This success is almost certainly due to the continual destruction of rectal adenomas as they arise. The question may, therefore, be asked, "Would the destruction of adenomas in nonpolyposis members of the general population also result in a similar decline in intestinal cancer?" The answer must surely be "yes." With the advent of colonoscopy and colonoscopic polypectomy new techniques are available for polyp control. At the same time information accumulates as to which individuals are at greatest risk of developing adenomatous polyps and to whom the new techniques can most effectively be applied. The combination of these circumstances suggests that a significant decrease in the incidence of cancer of the large bowel is now possible.

9
differential diagnosis

A number of conditions exist that are characterized by the formation of polyps in the gastrointestinal tract and that have at various times been confused with adenomatous polyposis (Bussey 1970). Most of these are distinguishable on clinical grounds and all but one on histological examination, which is of paramount importance for the correct treatment of gastrointestinal polyposis. Adenomatous polyposis, with its almost inevitably fatal outcome if untreated, is a serious disease, the diagnosis of which clinically and histologically is seldom in doubt. Incorrect diagnosis of other forms of polyposis may subject the patient to unnecessary surgery and possibly cause considerable anxiety to his relatives, when no inheritable factor is involved. In this connection it cannot be too strongly emphasized that, whenever possible, sample polyps should be removed for histological examination before treatment is undertaken. This may seem elementary, but reports have been published where neglect of this precaution has led to wrong treatment.

The main types of gastrointestinal polyposis are classified in Table 13.

1) Inflammatory Polyposis

a) Colitis polyposa.   In those countries where idiopathic proctocolitis is most frequently encountered, inflammatory polyposis is probably the most common type of intestinal polyposis to be found. The polyps may be surviving islands of inflamed mucosa (Fig. 47) or semidetached strips of mucous membrane, but mostly they are excrescences produced from these tags by partial or total healing during alternating periods of active and quiescent disease (Fig. 48). Microscopically the polyps are composed of varying proportions of intestinal epithelium, acute or chronic inflammatory cell aggregations, and fibrous tissue (Figs. 49 & 50). They may thus show a spectrum from acute inflammatory tissue without any epithelial element to completely healed fibrous mucosal tags. Inflammatory polyps are usually confined to the large intestine. The association

Table 13. Classification of different types of gastrointestinal polyposis

Inflammatory	Colitis polyposa Bilharzial polyposis Benign lymphoid polyposis
Hamartomatous	Peutz–Jeghers syndrome Multiple juvenile polyposis Neurofibromatous polyposis Lipomatous polyposis
Neoplastic	Adenomatous polyposis coli (including Gardner's syndrome) Minor or recessive adenomatous polyposis Lymphosarcomatous polyposis Leukemia polyposis
Miscellaneous	Metaplastic polyposis Cronkhite–Canada syndrome Pneumatosis cystoides intestinalis

of cancer of the colon and rectum with ulcerative colitis has now been established and it is not surprising if the occurrence of a malignant tumor and inflammatory polyps in a colon affected by ulcerative colitis is sometimes mistaken for adenomatous polyposis.

b) **Bilharzial polyposis.** Infestations with both Schistosoma mansoni and Schistosoma hemotobium may give rise to intestinal symptoms, particularly of the colon and rectum (Mehriz 1958; Pontes 1961; Medina et al. 1965). The intestinal lesions are hyperemia and edema of the mucosa, congestion or varicosity of the submucosal veins, ulceration, and polypoid tumors. The latter may be single or multiple and, since there is a familial tendency due to environment, such cases may be mistaken for polyposis coli. The polyps are easily distinguished from adenomas macroscopically, being more broad-based, often arising out of a swollen edematous mucosa, and having a ragged and inflamed appearance (Fig. 51). The histology is also different, as the polyps consist of irregular nonhyperplastic mucosal epithelium and edematous supporting stroma infiltrated with inflammatory cells and containing numerous parasites and ova (Fig. 52).

In those regions where bilharzia is endemic (Egypt, Central Africa, Brazil, Venezuela, and Puerto Rico) this form of polyploid disease of the intestine could be the one most commonly encountered. Cases have also been reported from China due to S. Japonica. Patients with polyposis coli, living in areas where bilharzia is endemic, may show evidence of both diseases.

c) **Multiple benign lymphoid polyps.** The gastrointestinal tract is a region rich in lymphoid tissue, owing to the presence of numerous

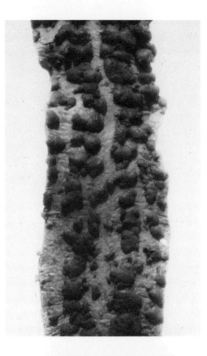

Fig. 47. Descending colon from a case of chronic ulcerative colitis. The dark "polyps" are inflamed tags of surviving mucous membrane standing out above the ulceration, which extends into the submucosa.

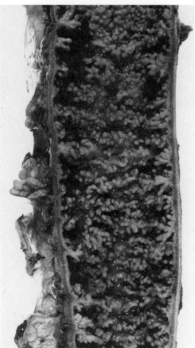

Fig. 48. Multiple polyps in a longstanding case of ulcerative colitis. The numerous pedunculated tumors are healed inflammatory polyps, though the naked-eye appearance of the specimen closely simulates that of polyposis coli.

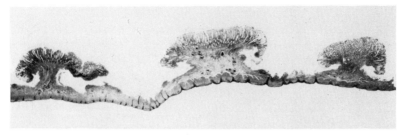

Fig. 49. Microscopic appearance of the wall of the colon in a case of ulcerative colitis. Three "polyps" are present, but these are islands of surviving mucosa undermined by the surrounding ulceration which extends down to the muscle coat. (×7) (Reduced by 30%)

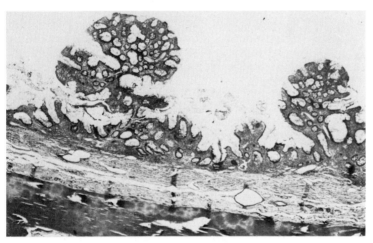

Fig. 50. Low power view of wall of colon showing ulcerative colitis in a quiescent stage. The mucosa is atrophic and irregular and two polyps are present. These consist of an overgrowth of epithelial tubules, sometimes cystic, irregularly arranged in a fibrous stroma. (×28) (Reduced by 30%)

lymphoid follicles and Peyer's patches. It is, therefore, not surprising that it is liable to become diffusely involved by inflammatory and neoplastic processes primarily concerned with lymphoid tissue. Multiple benign lymphoid polyps have already been referred to as not uncommon in the terminal ileum of polyposis coli patients. More extensive involvement of the small and large bowel is occasionally reported, particularly in children and young adults. Collins et al. (1966) published the case of a three-and-a-half-year-old child with many hundreds of lymphoid polyps throughout the colon, though the ileum was free. Louw (1968) recorded the occurrence of

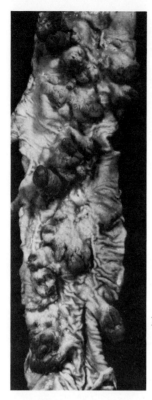

Fig. 51. Portion of the colon from a patient who died with schistosomiasis. The large polyps are composed of irregular mucosa and submucosa showing chronic inflammatory infiltration and fibrosis. Cysts filled with mucus, lymph, or cellular debris may be present.

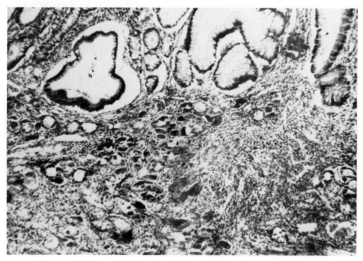

Fig. 52. High power view of one of the polyps shown in Fig. 51. Numerous bilharzial ova are present in the stroma of the tumor. (×80) (Reduced by 35%)

diffuse lymphoid polyps in three siblings. This type of lymphoid polyp is due to non-neoplastic hypertrophy resulting from inflammation or as a response to an immunological reaction. Gruenberg and Mackman (1972) report a case in a member of an adenomatous polyposis coli family, who underwent colectomy because of a radiological diagnosis of multiple polyps found subsequently to be of the lymphoid type.

d) **Other types of inflammatory polyposis.** Rarely, other types of inflammatory polyposis have been recorded, such as eosinophilic granulomatous polyposis (Legre et al. 1971), and in diffuse histoplasmosis (Bersack et al. 1958).

2) Hamartomatous Polyposis

a) **Peutz–Jeghers syndrome.** Though first described by Peutz in 1921, this disease received little attention until the publication of a paper by Jeghers et al. (1949). They reported the association of pigmented spots on the lips and buccal mucosa and, less commonly, the dorsal aspect of the hands and feet, with intestinal tumors producing intussusception and obstruction usually of the small intestine, though the polyps may be found in all parts of the gastrointestinal tract. The tumors can usually be numbered in dozens rather than hundreds and are never as numerous as adenomas in familial polyposis coli. They are composed of normal intestinal epithelium and smooth muscle in abnormal amounts and irregular arrangement (Figs. 53 & 54) and, therefore, are considered to be hamartomatous in nature. The smooth muscle element in the tumors differentiates them from the juvenile polyps that also may occur anywhere in the gastrointestinal tract and are also regarded as hamartomas. The disease is genetic and of a dominant character, though the full syndrome is not necessarily always manifested; some relatives of known cases may have pigmentation and no apparent polyps and others may have polyps with little or no buccal pigmentation.

Originally regarded as neoplastic lesions (they are still sometimes reported as benign "adenomas") with a high malignant potential, the recognition of Peutz–Jeghers polyps as hamartomas was linked with an absence of such potential. However, there are in the literature at least fifteen cases of definite cancer, mainly of the stomach and duodenum, in patients with the Peutz–Jeghers syndrome. Four other unpublished cases are known to exist (three in the St. Mark's Hospital Polyposis Register). Since, also, most of these cases were under 40 years of age, it would indicate that while the malignant potential of the syndrome is nothing like so serious as that of ade-

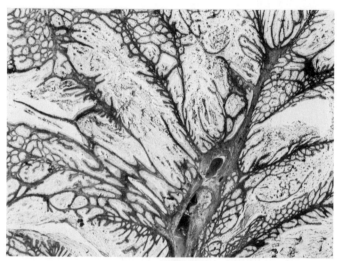

Fig. 53. Peutz–Jeghers polyp from the rectum. Villi lined by normal large intestinal epithelium are supported on a finely branching stroma consisting largely of smooth muscle fibers. (×14) (Reduced by 40%)

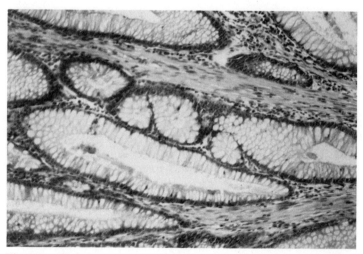

Fig. 54. High power view of a Peutz–Jeghers polyp showing the normal appearance of the epithelium and the smooth muscle element of the stroma. (×180) (Reduced by 40%)

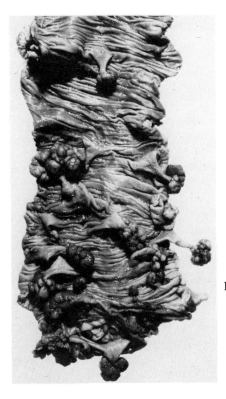

Fig. 55. Cecum and ascending colon from a boy aged 16 years who underwent colectomy for polyposis. Although most of the tumors resemble adenomas macroscopically, microscopic examination proved them to be juvenile polyps.

nomatous polyposis, it certainly cannot be ignored as negligible. Dodds et al. (1972) report a family in which eight members suffered from the Peutz–Jeghers syndrome and two of these also had carcinoma of the colon. This is probably the only record of such an association, but it should be noted that adenomas were also present, and it is more likely that the carcinomas arose in these rather than in the Peutz–Jeghers polyps.

b) **Multiple juvenile polyposis.** The condition known as multiple juvenile polyposis was first described by McColl et al. (1964) and elaborated upon by the same authors (Veale et al. 1966). Other authors had previously reported cases that were probably the same disease but were reported as adenomatosis (Wheeler 1926; Lefevre & Jacques 1951; El Sebai & Sobeih 1961). Coleman and Eckert (1956) did, however, refer to two examples, correctly diagnosing the tumors as juvenile polyps, but apparently without appreciating the significance of this observation, although they stated that the polyps were different from adenomas, were not precancerous, and did not necessarily require treatment by major surgery. The polyps are usually fewer in number than those of adenomatous polyposis (Fig. 55), and their distribution differs also in that they may be found anywhere in the gastrointestinal tract, though they are more common in the large intestine. The disease has a much earlier onset (the average is 6 years of age) than has polyposis coli, often being discovered in infancy and early childhood. The main clinical symptom is bleeding, associated usually with severe anemia, hypoproteinemia, malnutrition, and retarded development.

The polyps described in these earlier cases presented the histology of the juvenile or mucus-retention polyps found either singly or in small numbers in young children. They consisted of normal mucosal epithelium arranged in an irregular glandular pattern and surrounded by an increased amount of lamina propria (Fig. 56). The mucous glands sometimes become cystic and distended by mucus. Hemorrhage and secondary inflammation are often present. However, in some cases collected since the first eleven cases were reported the histology of the polyps has been more complex. Although a proportion of the tumors have shown the histology described above, i.e., that of juvenile polyps, others have been of a mixed or intermediate character between that of juvenile polyps and that of adenomas (Fig. 57). Definite adenomatous tumors have also been present in six patients with juvenile polyposis, and in one of these a rectal cancer has also been present. It has already been mentioned in Chapter 6, "Associated lesions," that the father of a young girl with juvenile polyposis was originally thought to have had adenomatous polyposis, but a further examination of the sections revealed that although some of these polyps were adenomas, others were juvenile, and the possibility that the two lesions can be associated in the same family is now less certain. Obviously, further research and observation are needed before deciding on the genetic relationships involved and in the malignant potentiality of juvenile polyposis.

Thirty-seven examples of multiple juvenile polyposis in twenty-eight families are now recorded in the St. Mark's Hospital Polyposis Register, including six families in which more than one member was affected. In one of these families (reported by Smilow et al. 1966) the disease appears in three generations.

Most of the cases have been solitary in character and not familial. Such patients have been observed to have a high incidence of other congenital abnormalities, such as malrotation of the bowel, heart lesions, hydrocephalus, etc., a feature that has been seen in only one affected member of the six families where more than one case has been found.

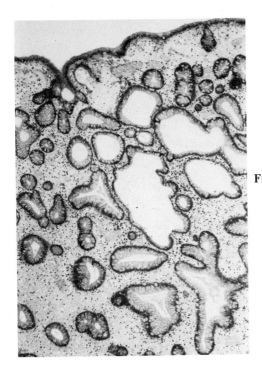

Fig. 56. Polyp from a patient with multiple juvenile polyposis. It consists of normal intestinal epithelium irregularly arranged in a stroma of lamina propria. Some of the tubules are cystic, due to retained mucus. The surface of the polyp is covered with a single cell layer of epithelial cells which is easily damaged, allowing secondary infection to take place. (×70) (Reduced by 40%)

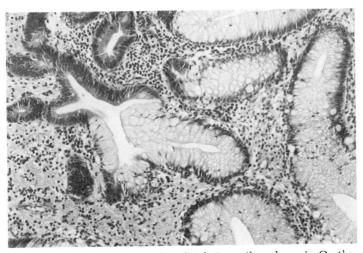

Fig. 57. Polyp from a case of multiple juvenile polyposis. On the right the appearances are those normally seen in a hamartomatous juvenile polyp, but on the left the epithelium shows hyperplasia with hyperchromatism, stratification, and other features that could be neoplastic in character. (×180) (Reduced by 40%)

MULTIPLE NEUROFIBROMATOSIS

Von Recklinghausen's disease (1882) is a genetic disease usually manifesting as multiple fibromas of the subcutaneous tissues, but occasionally associated with gastrointestinal neurofibromatosis. The intestinal lesions are usually present in the small intestine, but examples of colonic and rectal involvement have been reported (Levy & Khatib 1960; Gomez & Covelli 1961; Ghrist 1963). Microscopical examination of the intestinal tumors show them to be neurofibromas. More recently the occurrence of multiple mucosal neuromata in association with endocrine tumors has been observed by Williams and Pollock (1966), who consider this to be a syndrome allied to von Recklinghausen's disease. In an interesting case reported by Donnelly et al. (1969) multiple polyps in the large intestine were found to be a mixture of neurofibromas and juvenile polyps. It is also worth recording that a patient who underwent surgery for adenomatous polyposis at St. Mark's Hospital has subsequently been diagnosed as suffering from von Recklinghausen's disease.

LIPOMATOUS POLYPOSIS

Submucosal lipomas are not uncommon in the gastrointestinal tract, especially in the large intestine where they are either solitary or few in number. Rarely they may be multiple, as in the case reported by Ling et al. (1959), where numerous lipomas were present throughout the small and large intestines, and 195 cms of resected ileum and ascending colon contained 107 lipomas.

Lipomatosis may also occur in a more diffuse form when there is deposition of fat in the submucous coat of the colon and rectum, which gives an appearance of generalized polyposis due to the nodular mucosal surface (Swain et al. 1969). This unusual condition may be a result of malabsorption and is found only in young children.

NEOPLASTIC POLYPOSIS

"Minor" or "Recessive" Adenomatous Polyposis

Veale (1965) has postulated that three allelic genes may exist at the same locus; "x" the normal type and "P" and "p," both responsible for adenoma production. The former produces classical multiple polyposis coli and the latter only a few isolated adenomatous polyps, this being a recessive character only effective in the genotype "pp." If this theory is correct, the genotypes "Pp" and "Px" must exist, and this could explain why, whereas many patients present with advanced adenomatosis at an early age, others will not get symptoms until middle age or even later. It also takes into account the known facts of neoplastic disease of the large intestine, from the patient with a solitary adenoma or carcinoma and no family history, the families with two or three members with neoplasms of the intestinal tract, to the occasional family that is found to have a heavy incidence of bowel cancer.

The incidence rate of the "P" gene among births in this country has been estimated by Veale as about 1 in 24,000. He has also estimated that the proportions of the normal genotype "xx," the heterozygous "px," and the homozygous "pp" in the general population to be about 49%, 42%, and 9% respectively. The permutations of unions between these genotypes can give rise to varying proportions of the "pp" type in the families. Since these individuals will develop adenomas that may subsequently become malignant, it would be expected that in some families there will be an increased incidence of bowel cancer. This was in fact found to be the case when Lovett (1974) investigated the family history of patients with cancer of the large bowel. One-quarter of such patients were found to have at least one other relative with bowel cancer and an analysis of death certificates of family members revealed an incidence of intestinal cancer about five times greater than the expected rate.

With the possibility of two types of inherited adenomas of the large intestine, the problem arises of their differentiation and the often asked question, "How many polyps make polyposis?" A survey was carried out of all patients with adenomatous tumors seen at St. Mark's Hospital during the twelve-year period 1957–68. The number of adenomas found, both synchronously and metachronously, in each patient, excluding those with polyposis coli, is shown in Table 14. The majority of the patients had less than 6 polyps and there were only 25 of the 1,788 patients investigated who had 6 or more adenomas, the largest number being 48. Outside this particular series, patients with 60 or 70 adenomas have been occasionally encountered. If colonoscopy had been available at the time, the number of polyps would have been increased, but almost certainly only in the groups with fewest tumors. The patients with many adenomas were usually thoroughly investigated by multiple radiological examination and sometimes submitted to major surgery (Fig.

Table 14. Numerical distribution of adenomas among patients (St. Mark's Hospital 1957–68)

Number of adenomas	Number of patients	%
1	1,331	74.5
2	297	16.6
3	81	4.5
4	41	2.3
5	13	0.7
6	10	0.6
More than 6	15	0.8
TOTAL	1,788	100.0

58). It has already been shown that the average number of polyps in polyposis cases is about 1,000 and that it is rarely that less than 200 are present. The numerical distribution of adenomas per patient is shown diagrammatically in Fig. 59. The cases polarize into two groups corresponding with the recessive "pp" type and the dominant "P" or adenomatous polyposis coli type, and it seems reasonable to suggest that the figure of 100 adenomas makes a convenient practical division between them.

The patient with 50 or 60 adenomas frequently has a family history of bowel cancer, and it is not surprising that such cases are often thought to have polyposis coli. A few were originally included in the St. Mark's Hospital Polyposis Register, but subsequently removed. It is significant that so far no case of true adenomatous polyposis has been found in any relative of a patient with less than 100 polyps. Such a combination is not, however, impossible, as both types of inheritance could occur in one family, as is demonstrated in the pedigree below.

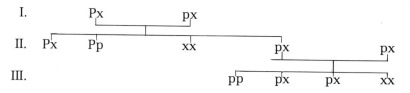

In generations I and II both genotypes "Px" and "Pp" would develop polyposis. The genotypes "px" and "xx" are not liable to produce even the odd polyp, but "pp" in generation III could produce some adenomas and possibly die from intestinal cancer. In such an event this case might be included erroneously in the pedigree as suffering from polyposis.

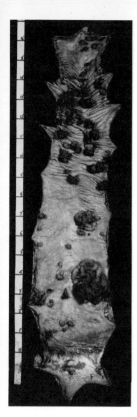

Fig. 58. Sigmoid colon and rectum removed by combined excision from a man aged 55 years. About 40 pedunculated and sessile tumors are present. Barium enema examination did not reveal any other tumors in the retained colon, and the patient survived for 25 years without further intestinal symptoms. There was no family history of bowel disease.

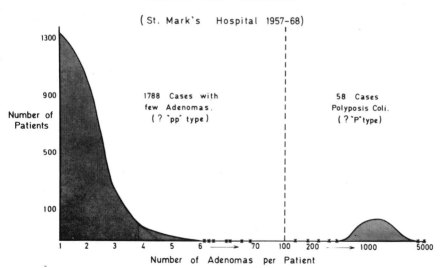

PATIENTS WITH ADENOMAS

(St. Mark's Hospital 1957–68)

1788 Cases with few Adenomas. (? "pp" type)

58 Cases Polyposis Coli. (? "P" type)

Fig. 59. Diagram showing the number of adenomas per patient. The figure of 100 adenomas is suggested as a practical division between the recessive type ("pp") and the dominant type ("P") of inherited adenomas as postulated in Veale's hypothesis. (It should be noted that owing to the wide variation in both the number of adenomas and of patients the scale has been distorted to accommodate the graph.)

LYMPHOSARCOMATOUS AND LEUKEMIC POLYPOSIS

Lymphosarcoma of the intestine is usually a solitary lesion, but may take the form of widespread polyps formed by submucosal deposits of malignant tissue in the lymphoid follicles (Fig. 60) (Cornes 1961; Poutasse 1963; Pochaczevsky & Sherman 1962). The barium enema studies of such cases may well suggest a diagnosis of multiple adenomatosis, though biopsy of a polyp would quickly correct this misconception (Fig. 61).

Finally, it may be mentioned that a case of chronic lymphatic leukemia has been known to present initially with intestinal symptoms. On sigmoidoscopy multiple polypoid tumors were found in the rectum, and a tentative diagnosis of polyposis coli was considered. However, operation was delayed and the rapid deterioration in the patient's condition led to the correct diagnosis being established.

MISCELLANEOUS TYPES OF POLYPOSIS

Multiple Metaplastic Polyps

Schmieden and Westhues (1927) first described the tumors commonly found in the large intestine, to which they gave the name "hyperplastic polyps." These are sessile button-like tumors, seldom more than 0.5 cms in diameter and paler in color than the surrounding mucosa. Occasionally the tumors may be as large as 2.0 cms in diameter and are then polypoid in appearance. They are symptomless and are incidental findings in routine examinations. Microscopically the metaplastic polyps show a decrease in the number of epithelial cells, which are of irregular height with uneven staining nuclei. There is loss of mucus secretion and replacement of goblet cells by absorptive cells, these changes being more noticeable in the upper part of the crypts (Figs. 62 & 63). Westhues (1934) recognized the tumors to be different from adenomas and "harmless" in not sharing the premalignant character of the adenoma. Morson (1962b) found no evidence of hyperplasia in the tumors and called them "metaplastic," as indicative of the differing histological appearance, the term being also noncommittal as to the cause. The widespread incidence of metaplastic polyps has been pointed out by Arthur (1962; 1968). They appear to be confined to the large intestine and are most common in the rectum. In rare instances they may be so numerous and unusually large as to be mistaken for polyposis coli

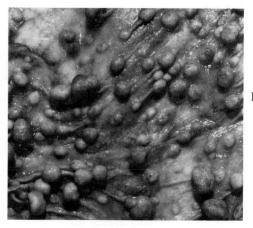

Fig. 60. Multiple lymphosarcomatous polyps of the sigmoid colon. The lesions, which originate in the submucosa, are usually covered with intact mucosa, giving them a smooth surface in contrast to the lobulated, fissured appearance of adenomas.

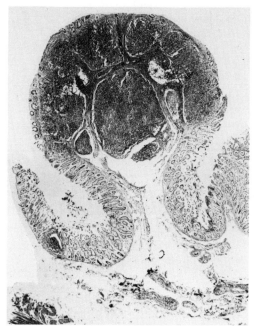

Fig. 61. Lymphosarcomatous polyp from the colon shown in Fig. 60. The tumor is composed of lymphoid tissue lacking the normal follicular pattern. A layer of attenuated mucosa is stretched over the lesion, forming a smooth surface. (×18) (Reduced by 40%)

(Fig. 64). Six cases of this nature have been recorded in the St. Mark's Hospital Polyposis Register. Sometimes there is an associated history of intestinal cancer, either in the patient or his relatives, which increases the tendency to confuse the lesion with adenomatous polyposis. However, care has to be exercised in dismissing the condition as only metaplastic polyposis, as adenomas are sometimes present among the metaplastic polyps.

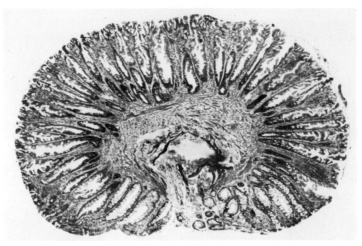

Fig. 62. Metaplastic polyp from the rectum. Although there is some epithelial hyperplasia in the lower part of the crypts, elsewhere there is a decrease in the number of epithelial cells, which are of irregular height with uneven staining nuclei. The loss of mucus secretion and the replacement of goblet cells by absorptive cells is most noticeable in the upper part of the crypts. (×60) (Reduced by 40%)

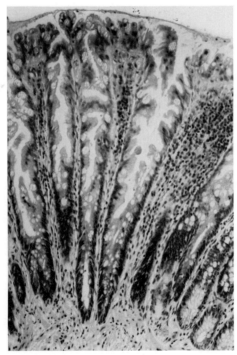

Fig. 63. Part of the metaplastic (hyperplastic) polyp shown in Figure 62. There is great irregularity in the size of the epithelial cells, with loss of goblet cells, these features being more marked in the upper half of the tubules. (×180) (Reduced by 40%)

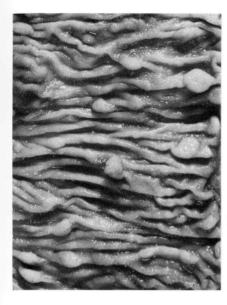

Fig. 64. Close-up photograph of colon removed for suspected adenomatous polyposis. Histological examination showed the polyps to be metaplastic (hyperplastic) in character.

Cronkhite–Canada Syndrome

The association of gastrointestinal polypi, alopecia, and nail dystrophy was first reported by Cronkhite and Canada (1955); since then about seven or eight further individual case reports have been made (Johnson et al. 1962; Jarnum & Jensen 1966; Gill & Wilkin 1967). The intestinal symptoms are mainly diarrhea and increased fecal fat. The general impression is that the disease is of the malabsorption-vitamin deficiency type, similar to pellagra, and has a poor prognosis. The polyps may occur in any part of the gastrointestinal tract and take the form of cystic degeneration of the mucosa with secondary inflammatory changes similar to those previously reported as "colitis cystica superficialis." At least one case was thought to be ulcerative colitis, with extensive pseudopolyposis, and was treated by total proctocolectomy (Ryall 1966).

Pneumatosis Cystoides Intestinalis

In this condition gas-filled cysts are present in the submucosa of the colon, particularly the left colon, and form polypoid swellings of the mucosal surface, which are apt to be mistaken for multiple adenomatosis on barium enema examination of the large intestine. The cysts usually have thin fibrous walls with no epithelial lining, and their etiology is still undecided. The real nature of the "tumors" is obvious on histological examination.

references

ABRAMSON, D. J. "Multiple polyposis in children: A review and a report of a case of a 6-year-old child who had associated nephrosis and asthma." *Surgery* 61 (1967): 288–301.

ALM, T. and Licznerski, G. "The intestinal polyposes." *Clins. Gastroent.* 2 (1973): 577–602.

ARTHUR, J. F. "The significance of small mucosal polyps of the rectum." *Proc.Roy.Soc.Med.* 55 (1962): 703.

ARTHUR, J. F. "Structure and significance of metaplastic nodules in the rectal mucosa." *J.clin.Path.* 21 (1968): 735–43.

BACON, H. E., Giambalvo, G. P., Sauer, I., Fleming, J. P., and Villalba, G. "Intestinal polyposis." *J.internat.Coll.Surg.* 28 (1957): 346–56.

BARTHOLOMEW, L. G., and Dahlin, D. C. "Intestinal polyposis and mucocutaneous pigmentation (Peutz–Jeghers syndrome). Further comments and report of an additional case." *Minnesota Med.* 41 (1958): 848–52.

BERSACK, S. R., Howe, J. S., and Rabson, A. S. "Inflammatory pseudopolyposis of the small and large intestines with the Peutz–Jeghers syndrome in a case of diffuse histoplasmosis." *Amer.J.Roentgenol.* 80 (1958): 73–78.

BICKERSTETH, R. A. "Multiple polypi of the rectum occurring in a mother and child." *St.Bartholomew's Hosp.Rep.* 26 (1890): 299.

BIRBECK, M. S. C., and Dukes, C. E. "Electron microscopy of rectal neoplasms." *Proc.Roy.Soc.Med.* 56 (1963): 793–98.

BIRKETT, D. P., "Epidemiology of cancer of the colon and rectum." *Cancer* 28 (1971): 3–13.

BREMNER, C. G. "Ano-rectal disease in the South African Bantu—III carcinoma of the rectum." *S.Afr.J.Surg.* 3 (1965): 35–40.

BUSSEY, H. J. R. "The long-term results of surgical treatment of cancer of the rectum." *Proc.Roy.Soc,Med.* 56 (1963): 494–96.

BUSSEY, H. J. R. "Gastrointestinal polyposis." *Gut* 11 (1970): 970–78.

BUSSEY, H. J. R. "Extracolonic lesions associated with polyposis coli." *Proc. Roy.Soc.Med.* 65 (1972): 294.

BUSSEY, H. J. R., Dukes, C. E., and Lockhart–Mummery, H. E. "Cancer of the rectum," in *Monographs on Neoplastic Diseases at Various Sites*, Vol. 3, Chap. 23, ed. C. E. Dukes. Edinburgh and London: E. & S. Livingstone, 1960.

BUSSEY, H. J. R., Wallace, M. H., and Morson, B. C. "Metachronous carcinoma of the large intestine and intestinal polyps." *Proc.Roy.Soc.Med.* 60 (1967): 208–10.

CABOT, R. C. "Case records of the Massachusetts General Hospital, Case No. 21061." *New Engl.J.Med.* 212 (1935): 263–67.

CAMIEL, M. R., Mulé, J. E., Alexander, L. L., and Benninghoff, D. L. "Association of thyroid carcinoma with Gardner's syndrome in siblings." *New Engl. J.Med.* 278 (1968): 1058–59.

CAPPS, W. F., Jr., Lewis, M. I., and Gazzaniga, D. A. "Carcinoma of the colon, ampulla of Vater and urinary bladder associated with familial multiple polyposis." *Dis.Colon Rect.* 11 (1968): 298–305.

CHARGELAIGUE, A. "Des polypes du rectum." Thesis, Paris, 1859.

CHIAT, H., Ross, S. T., Janelli, D. E., and Mandel, P. R. "Familial polyposis of the colon with subsequent development of a duodenal polyp. Report of a case." *Dis.Colon Rect.* 5 (1962): 444–45.

COLCOCK, B. P., and Zomorodian, A. A. "Gardner's syndrome. Multiple polyposis of colon, bone tumours and soft-tissue tumours." *Postgrad.Med.* 40 (1966): 29–34.

COLE, J. W., and Holden, W. D. "Postcolectomy regression of adenomatous polyps of the rectum." *Arch.Surg.* 79 (1959): 385–92.

COLE, J. W., and McKalen, A. "Studies on the morphogenesis of adenomatous polyps in the human colon." *Cancer* 16 (1963): 998–1002.

COLE, J. W., McKalen, A. and Powell, J. "The rôle of the ileal contents in the spontaneous regression of rectal adenomas." *Dis.Colon Rect.* 4 (1961): 413–18.

COLEMAN, S. T., and Eckert, C. "Preservation of rectum in familial polyposis of the colon and rectum." *Arch.Surg.* 73 (1956): 635–44.

COLLINS, J. O., Falk, M., and Guibone, R. "Benign lymphoid polyposis of the colon." *Pediatrics* 38 (1966): 897–99.

CORNES, J. S. "Multiple lymphomatous polyposis of the gastrointestinal tract." *Cancer* 14 (1961): 249–57.

CORVISART, L. "Hypertrophie partielle de la muqueuse intestinale." *Bull. Soc.Anat.* 22 (1847): 400.

CRAIL, H. W. "Multiple primary malignancies arising in rectum, brain and thyroid." *U.S. Navy Med.Bull.* 49 (1949): 123–28.

CRIPPS, W. H. "Two cases of disseminated polypus of the rectum." *Trans.path. Soc.Lond.* 33 (1882): 165–68.

CRONKHITE, L. W., and Canada, W. J. "Generalised gastro-intestinal polyposis. Unusual syndrome of polyposis, pigmentation, alopecia and onychotrophia." *New Engl.J.Med.* 252 (1955): 1011.

DEVIC, A., and Bussy, M. M. "Un cas de polypose adenomateuse généralisée à tout l'intestin." *Arch.Mal.App.dig.* 6 (1912): 278–89.

DODDS, W. J., Schulte, W. J., Hensley, G. T., and Hogan, W. J. "Peutz–Jeghers syndrome and gastrointestinal malignancy." *Amer.J.Roentgenol.* 115 (1972): 374–77.

DONNELLY, W. H., Sieber, W. K., and Yunis, E. J. "Polypoid ganglioneurofibromatosis of the large bowel." *Arch.Path.* 87 (1969): 537–41.

DORMANDY, T. L. "Medical progress: gastro-intestinal polyposis with mucocutaneous pigmentation (Peutz–Jeghers syndrome)." *New Engl.J.Med.* 256 (1957): 1093, 1141, 1186.

DRASAR, B. S., and Hill, M. J. "Intestinal bacteria and cancer." *Amer.J.clin. Nutr.* 25 (1972): 1399–1404.

DUHAMEL, J., Berthon, G., and Dubarry, J. J. "Étude mathématique de l'hérédité de la polypose recto-colique." *J.Génét.Hum.* 9 (1960): 65–77.

DUKES, C. E. "The hereditary factor in polyposis intestine or multiple adenomata." *Cancer Rev.* 5 (1930): 241–56.

DUKES, C. E. "The classification of cancer of the rectum." *J.Path.Bact.* 35 (1932): 323.

DUKES, C. E. "An explanation of the difference between a papilloma and an adenoma of the rectum." *Proc.Roy.Soc.Med.* 40 (1947): 829–30.

DUKES, C. E. "Familial intestinal polyposis." *Ann.Eugen.Lond.* 17 (1952): 1–29.

DUNNING, E. J., and Ibrahim, K. S. "Gardner's syndrome: report of a case." *Ann.Surg.* 161 (1965): 565–68.

EL SEBAI, I., and Sobeih, A. "Sarcoidosis, endometriosis and polyposis of the colon and rectum." *Kasr-El-Aini J.Surg.* 2 (1961): 848–67.

EVERSON, T. C., and Allen, M. J. "Subtotal colectomy with ileosigmoidostomy and fulguration of polyps in retained colon: Evaluation as method of treatment of polyposis (adenomatous) of colon." *Arch.Surg.* 69 (1954): 806–17.

FISHER, E. R., and Sharkey, D. A. "The ultrastructure of colonic polyps and cancer with special reference to the epithelial inclusion bodies of Leuchtenberger." *Cancer* 15 (1962): 160–70.

FITZGERALD, G. M. "Multiple composite odontomas coincidental with other tumorous conditions. Report of a case." *J.Amer.Dent.Ass.* 30 (1943): 1408–17.

FLOTTE, C. T., O'Dell, F. C., Jr., and Coller, F. A. "Polyposis of the colon." *Ann.Surg.* 144 (1956): 165–69.

GARDNER, E. J. "A genetic and clinical study of intestinal polyposis, a predisposing factor for carcinoma of the colon and rectum." *Amer.J.hum.Genet.* 3 (1951): 167–76.

GARDNER, E. J. "Follow-up study of a family group exhibiting dominant inheritance for a syndrome including intestinal polyps, osteomas, fibromas and epidermal cysts." *Amer.J.hum.Genet.* 14 (1962): 376–90.

GARDNER, E. J. "Gardner's syndrome re-evaluated after twenty years." *Proc. Utah Academy* 46 (1969): 1–11.

GARDNER, E. J., and Plenk, H. P. "Hereditary pattern for multiple osteomas in a family group." *Amer.J.hum.Genet.* 4 (1952): 31–36.

GARDNER, E. J., and Richards, R. C. "Multiple cutaneous and sub-cutaneous lesions occurring simultaneously with hereditary polyposis and osteomatosis." *Amer.J.hum.Genet.* 5 (1953): 139–47.

GHRIST, T. D. "Gastrointestinal involvement in neurofibromatosis." *Arch. Intern.Med.* 112 (1963): 357–62.

GIBBS, N. M. "Incidence and significance of argentaffin and Paneth cells in some tumours of the large intestine." *J.clin.Path.* 20 (1967): 826–31.

GILL, W., and Wilkin, B. J. "Diffuse gastrointestinal polyposis associated with hypoproteinaemia." *J.Roy.Coll.Surg.Edinb.* 12 (1967): 149–56.

GOMEZ, M. A., and Covelli, J. R. "Colonic and rectal manifestations of Recklinghausen's disease." *Rev.méd.Chile* 89 (1961): 1070–71.

GORDON, W. C., Jr., Rast, M. F., and Whelan, T. J., Jr. "Gardner's syndrome." *Ann.Surg.* 155 (1962): 538–42.

GORLIN, R. J., and Chaudhry, A. P. "Multiple osteomatosis, fibromas, lipomas and fibrosarcomas of the skin and mesentery, epidermoid inclusion cysts of the skin, leiomyomas and multiple intestinal polyposis." *New Engl.J.Med.* 263 (1960): 1151–58.

GRINNELL, R. S., and Lane, N. "Benign and malignant adenomatous polyps and papillary adenomas of the colon and rectum. An analysis of 1,856 tumors in 1,335 patients." *Surg.Gynec.Obstet.* 106 (1958): 519–38.

GRUENBERG, J., and Mackman, S. "Multiple lymphoid polyps in familial polyposis." *Ann.Surg.* 175 (1972): 552–54.

HAENSZEL, W., and Kurihara, M. "Studies of Japanese migrants. I. Mortality from cancer and other diseases among Japanese in the United States." *J.Nat. Cancer Inst.* 40 (1968): 43–68.

HANDFORD, H. "Disseminated polypi of the large intestine becoming malignant." *Trans.path.Soc.Lond.* 41 (1890): 133.

HAYES H. T., Burr, H. B., and Melton, W. T. "Management of adenomatosis or polyposis of the colon and rectum: report of 5 cases." *Texas State J.Med.* 55 (1959): 894–97.

HEALD, R. J. "Gardner's syndrome in association with two tumours in the ileum." *Proc.Roy.Soc.Med.* 60 (1967): 914–15.

HILL, M. J., Drasar, B. S., Aries, V., Crowther, J. S., Hawksworth, G., and Williams, R. E. O. "Bacteria and aetiology of cancer of the large bowel." *Lancet* 1 (1971): 95–100.

HOFFMANN, D. C., and Goligher, J. C. "Polyposis of the stomach and small intestine in association with familial polyposis coli." *Brit.J.Surg.* 58 (1971): 126–28.

HUBBARD, T. B. "Familial polyposis of the colon: the fate of the retained rectum after colectomy in children." *Amer.Surgeon* 23 (1957): 577–86.

HUTCHINSON, J. "Pigmentation of lips and mouth." *Arch.Surg.Lond.* 7 (1896): 290.

JARNUM, S., and Jensen, H. "Diffuse gastrointestinal polyposis with ectodermal changes." *Gastroenterology* 50 (1966): 107–18.

JEGHERS, H., McKusick, V. A., and Katz, K. H. "Generalized intestinal polyposis and melanin spots of the oral mucosa, lips and digits." *New Engl.J.Med.* 241 (1949): 993–1005.

JOHNSON, M. M., Vosburgh, J. W., Wiens, A. T., and Walsh, G. C. "Gastrointestinal polyposis associated with alopecia, pigmentation and atrophy of the fingernails and toenails." *Ann.intern.Med.* 56 (1962): 935–40.

KAPLAN, B. J. "Gardner's syndrome: heredo-familial adenomatosis associated with 'soft and hard' fibrous tumors and epidermoid cysts." *Dis.Colon Rect.* 4 (1961): 252–62.

KIM, C. E., and Kim, M. J. "Familial polyposis coli: a case report and review of the literature." *J.Korea Surg.Soc.* 8 (1966): 51–55.

KNAPP, G. M. "Diffuse polyposis of the colon." *Rocky Mountain med.J.* 62 (1965): 36–37.

KODAIRA, T. "Clinical observations of total colectomy in Japan." *Dis.Colon Rect.* 7 (1964): 424–27.

LANE, N., and Lev, R. "Observations on the origin of adenomatous epithelium of the colon: serial section studies of minute polyps in familial polyposis." *Cancer* 16 (1963): 751–64.

LAQUEUR, G. L. "The induction of intestinal neoplasms in rats with the glycoside cycasin and its aglycone." *Virchows Arch.path.Anat.* 340 (1965): 151–63.

LEBERT, H. "Traité d'Anatomie pathol." Paris, 1861. Quoted by Hewitt and Howard (1915).

LEFEVRE, H. W., and Jacques, T. F. "Multiple polyposis in an infant of four months." *Amer.J.Surg.* 81 (1951): 90–91.

LEGRE, M., Saint-Pierre, A., and Gratecos, N. "Granulome eosinophile rectocolique diffus a expansions polypoides multiple; étude clinique, radiologique, endoscopique et histologique d'un cas." *Ann.Gastroenterol. Hepatol.* 7 (1971): 429–39.

LEPPARD, B. "Epidermoid cysts and polyposis coli." *Proc.Roy.Soc.Med.* 67 (1974): 1036–37.

LEUCHTENBERGER, C. "Cytoplasmic 'inclusion bodies' containing desoxyribose nucleic acid (DNA) in cells of human rectal polyps." *Lab.Invest.* 3 (1954): 132–42.

LEUCHTENBERGER, C., Leuchtenberger, R., and Liebv, E. "Studies of cytoplasmic inclusions containing desoxyribose nucleic acid (DNA) in human rectal polypoid tumours including familial hereditary type." *Acta genet. et statist.med.* 6 (1956): 291–97.

LEVY, D., and Khatib, R. "Intestinal neurofibromatosis with malignant degeneration: report of a case." *Dis.Colon Rect.* 3 (1960): 140–44.

LING, C. S., Leagus, C., and Stahlgren, L. H. "Intestinal lipomatosis." *Surgery* 46 (1959): 1054–59.

LOCKHART–MUMMERY, H. E. "Intestinal polyposis: the present position." *Proc.Roy.Soc.Med.* 60 (1967): 381–88.

LOCKHART–MUMMERY, J. P. "Cancer and heredity." *Lancet* 1 (1925): 427–29.

LOUW, J. H. "Polypoid lesions of the large bowel in children with particular reference to benign lymphoid polyposis." *Pediatric Surgery* 3 (1968): 195–209.

LOVETT, E. "Familial factors in the etiology of carcinoma of the bowel." *Proc.Roy.Soc.Med.* 67 (1974): 751–52.

LUSCHKA, H. *Virchow's Arch.f.pathol.Anat.* 20 (1861): 133. (Quoted by Hewitt and Howard, 1915.)

MARSHALL, W. H., Martin, F. I. R., and Mackay, I. R. "Gardner's syndrome with adrenal carcinoma." *Aust.Ann.Med.* 16 (1967): 242–44.

McADAM, W. A. F., and Goligher, J. C. "The occurrence of desmoids in patients with familial polyposis coli." *Brit.J.Surg.* 57 (1970): 618–31.

McCOLL, I., Bussey, H. J. R., Veale, A. M. O., and Morson, B. C. "Juvenile polyposis coli." *Proc.Roy.Soc.Med.* 57 (1964): 896–97.

MACDONALD, J. M., Davis, W. C., Crago, H. R., and Berk, A. D. "Gardner's syndrome and peri-ampullary malignancy." *Amer.J.Surg.* 113 (1967): 425–30.

McFARLAND, P. H., Jr., Scheetz, W. L., and Knisley, R. E. "Gardner's syndrome: report of two families." *J.oral Surg.* 26 (1968): 632–38.

McKENNEY, D. C. "Multiple polyposis of colon: familial factor and malignant tendency." *J.Amer.med.Ass.* 107 (1936): 1871–76.

McKENNEY, D. C. "Multiple polyposis: congenital, heredofamilial, malignant." *Amer.J.Surg.* 46 (1939): 204–16.

McKUSICK, V. A. "Genetic factors in intestinal polyposis." *J.Amer.med.Ass.* 182 (1962): 271–77.

McQUAIDE, J. R., and Stewart, A. W. "Familial polyposis of the colon in the Bantu." *S.Afr.med.J.* 46 (1972): 1241–46.

MEDINA, J. T., Seaman, W. B., Guzman–Acosta, C., and Diaz–Bonnet, R. B. "The roentgen appearance of Schistosomiasis Mansoni involving the colon." *Radiology* 85 (1965): 682–88.

MEHRIZ, I. "Bilharziasis of the colon." *Kasr-El-Aini Gazette* 24 (1958): 207–19.

MENZEL, D. *Acta Medicorum Berlinensium* 9 (1721): 78. Quoted by Hewitt and Howard (1915).

MOERTEL, C. G., Hill, J. R., and Adson, M. A. "Surgical management of multiple polyposis." *Arch.Surg.* 100 (1970): 521–26.

MORSON, B. C. "Some peculiarities in the histology of intestinal polyps." *Dis.Colon Rect.* 5 (1962a): 337–44.

MORSON, B. C. "Precancerous lesions of the colon and rectum." *J.Amer.med. Ass.* 179 (1962b): 316–21.

MORSON, B. C. "Factors influencing the prognosis of early cancer of the rectum." *Proc.Roy.Soc.Med.* 59 (1966): 607–8.

MORSON, B. C. "Precancerous and early malignant lesions of the large intestine." *Brit.J.Surg.* 55 (1968): 725–31.

MORSON, B. C. "The polyp-cancer sequence in the large bowel." *Proc.Roy. Soc.Med.* 67 (1974): 451–57.

MORSON, B. C., and Bussey, H. J. R. "Predisposing causes of intestinal cancer," in *Current Problems in Surgery*, Chicago: Year Book Medical Publishers, 1970.

NEEL, J. V. "Problems in the estimation of the frequency of uncommon inherited traits." *Amer.J.hum.Genet.* 6 (1954): 51.

NIEMACK, J. "Intestinal polyposis and carcinoma." *Ann.Surg.* 36 (1902): 104.

NISHIMURA, M., et al. "A case of familial polyposis." *Surg.Ther.* (Osaka) 21 (1969): 488–92.

PARKS, T. G., Bussey, H. J. R., and Lockhart–Mummery, H. E. "Familial polyposis coli associated with extracolonic abnormalities." *Gut* 11 (1970): 323–29.

PEUTZ, J. L. A. "Over een zeer merkwaardige gecombineerde familiaire polyposis van de slijmvliezen van den tractus intestinalis met die van de neuskeelholte en gepaard met eigenaardige pigmentaties van huid en slijmvliezen." *Nederl.maandschr.voor Geneesk* 10 (1921): 134–46.

PIERCE, E. R. "Some genetic aspects of familial multiple polyposis of the colon in a kindred of 1,422 members." *Dis.Colon Rect.* 11 (1968): 321–29.

POCHACZEVSKY, R., and Sherman, R. S. "Diffuse lymphomatous disease of the colon: its roentgen appearance." *Amer.J.Roentgenol.* 87 (1962): 670–84.

PONTES, J. H. "Rectosigmoidoscopic aspects of Mansonian schistosomiasis in Brazil." *Dis.Colon Rect.* 4 (1961): 343–48.

POUTASSE, J. D. "Unusual colon manifestations of lymphosarcoma." *Amer. J.dig.Dis.* 8 (1963): 545–56.

RECIO, P., and Bussey, H. J. R. "The pathology and prognosis of carcinoma of the rectum in the young." *Proc.Roy.Soc.Med.* 58 (1965): 789–90.

REED, T. E., and Neel, J. V. "A genetic study of multiple polyposis of the colon (with an appendix deriving a method of estimating relative fitness)." *Amer. J.hum.Genet.* 7 (1955): 236–63.

RINTALA, A. "Histological appearance of gastrointestinal polyps in Peutz–Jeghers syndrome." *Acta chir.scand.* 117 (1959): 366–73.

ROKITANSKY, C. "Der dysenterische prozess auf dem dickdarm." *Med.Jahrb. des K.K. öst Staates* 29 (1839): 88.

RYALL, R. J. "Polypoid hypertrophy of the gastrointestinal mucosa presenting as ulcerative colitis." *Proc.Roy.Soc.Med.* 59 (1966): 614–15.

SCARBOROUGH, R. A. "Management of polyps of the large bowel." *Southern med.J.* 58 (1955): 455–58.

SCARBOROUGH, R. A., and Klein, R. R. "Polypoid lesions of colon and rectum." *Amer.J.Surg.* 76 (1948): 723–27.

SCHAUPP, W. C., and Volpe, P. A. "Management of diffuse colonic polyposis." *Amer.J.Surg.* 124 (1972): 218–22.

SCHMIEDEN, Y., and Westhues, H. "Zur klinik und pathologie der dickdarm-polypen und deren klinischen und pathologisch anatomischen beziehungen dickdarmkarzinom." *Deutsch.Ztschr.f.Chir.* 202 (1927): 1.

SHEPHERD, J. A. "Familial polyposis of the colon with associated connective tissue tumours." *J.Roy.Coll.Surg. Edinb.* 4 (1958): 31–38.

SIMPSON, R. D., Harrison, E. G., and Mayo, C. W. "Mesenteric fibromatosis in familial polyposis: a variant of Gardner's syndrome." *Cancer* 17 (1924): 526–34.

SMIDDY, F. G., and Goligher, J. C. "Results of surgery in treatment of cancer of the large intestine." *Brit.med.J.* 1 (1957): 793.

SMILOW, P. C., Pryor, C. A., Jr., and Swinton, N. W. "Juvenile polyposis coli: a report of three patients in three generations of one family." *Dis.Colon Rect.* 9 (1966): 248–54.

SMITH, W. G. "Desmoid tumours in familial multiple polyposis." *Mayo Clin.Proc.* 34 (1959): 31–38.

SMITH, W. G. "Familial multiple polyposis: research tool for investigating the etiology of carcinoma of the colon?" *Dis.Colon Rect.* 11 (1968): 17–31.

SPJUT, H. J., and Noall, M. W. "Experimental induction of tumours of the large bowel in rats. A review of the experience with 3-2′ dimethyl-4-amino-biphenyl." *Cancer* 28 (1971): 29–37.

SWAIN, V. A. J., Young, W. F., and Pringle, E. M. "Hypertrophy of the appendices epiploicae and lipomatous polyposis of the colon." *Gut* 10 (1969): 587–89.

THOMFORD, N. R., and Greenberger, N. J. "Lymphoid polyps of the ileum associated with Gardner's syndrome." *Arch.Surg.* 96 (1968): 289–91.

TURCOT, J., Despres, J. P. and St. Pierre, F. "Malignant tumours of the central nervous system associated with familial polyposis of the colon." *Dis.Colon Rect.* 2 (1959): 465–68.

UTSUNOMIYA, J., and Nakamura, T. "The occult osteomatous changes in the mandible in patients with familial polyposis coli." *Brit. J. Surg.* 62 (1975): 45–51.

VEALE, A. M. O. "Possible autosomal linkage in man." *Nature* 182 (1958): 409–10.

VEALE, A. M. O. "Intestinal polyposis." Eugenics Laboratory Memoirs Series 40. London: 1965. Cambridge University Press.

VEALE, A. M. O., McColl, I., Bussey, H. J. R., and Morson, B. C. "Juvenile polyposis coli." *J.med.Genet.* 3 (1966): 5–16.

VIRCHOW, R. *Die krankhaften Geschwülste.* Berlin: A. Hirschwald, 1863.

VON RECKLINGHAUSEN, F. *Uber die multiplen fibrome der haut und ihre beziehung zu den multiplen neuromen.* Berlin: A. Hirschwald, 1882.

WAGNER, J. "Einige formen von darmgeschwüren: (3) die dysenterische darmverschwürung." *Med.Jahrb.des k.k. öst Staates* 11 (1832): 274.

WALB, D., and Sandritter, W. "Inclusion bodies in rectal polyps." *Arch.Path.* 78 (1964): 104–7.

WELIN, S., Youker, J., Spratt, J. S., Linnell, F., Spjut, H. J., Johnson, R. E., and Ackerman, L. V. "The rates and patterns of growth of 375 tumours of the large intestine and rectum observed serially by double contrast enema study (Malmö technique)." *Amer.J.Roentgen.* 90 (1963): 673–87.

WENCKERT, A. "Cancer of the colon and rectum." *Acta chir. scand. Suppl.* 332 (1965): 73–79.

WESTHUES, H. "Die pathologisch-anatomischen grundlagen der chirugie des rectumkarzinomas." *Georg Thieme*, Leipzig (1934).

WESTON, S. D., and Weiner, M. "Familial polyposis associated with a new type of soft-tissue lesion (skin pigmentation): report of three cases and a review of the literature." *Dis.Colon Rect.* 10 (1967): 311–21.

WHEELER, W. I. de C. "Multiple polypi of the colon." *Brit.J.Surg.* 14 (1926): 58–66.

WILLIAMS, E. D., and Pollock, D. J. "Multiple mucosal neuromata with endocrine tumours: a syndrome allied to von Recklinghausen's disease." *J.Path. Bact.* 91 (1966): 71–80.

WOODWARD, J. J. "Pseudo-polypi of the colon: an anomalous result of follicular ulceration." *Amer.J.med.Sci.* 81 (1881): 142.

WYNDER, E. L., Kajitani, T., Ishikawa, S., Dodo, H., and Takano, A. "Environmental factors of cancer of the colon and rectum. II. Japanese epidemiological data." *Cancer* 23 (1969): 1210–20.

ZAHLMANN, S. "Polyposis intestini crassi." *Hospitals Tidende* 11 (1903): 1267–74.

index